AROMATHERAPY FOR LIFE EMPOWERMENT

USING ESSENTIAL OILS TO ENHANCE BODY, MIND, SPIRIT WELL-BEING

DAVID SCHILLER & CAROL SCHILLER

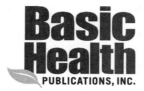

Basic Health

PUBLICATIONS, INC.

The book is for educational purposes and is not intended to replace the services of a natural practitioner. Please read the Safety, Storage and Handling of Oils in Chapter 2: How To Use Aromatherapy before using any of the essential oils or formulas. The safe and proper use of the oils is the sole responsibility of the reader. The authors and publisher assume no responsibility or liability for anyone's misuse, carelessness, allergic reactions, skin sensitivity, or any other conditions arising directly or indirectly from the use of this book.

The publisher does not advocate the use of any particular healthcare protocol but believes the information in this book should be available to the public. The publisher and author are not responsible for any adverse effects or consequences resulting from the use of the suggestions, preparations, or procedures discussed in this book. Should the reader have any questions concerning the appropriateness of any procedures or preparation mentioned, the author and the publisher strongly suggest consulting a professional healthcare advisor.

Basic Health Publications, Inc.
28812 Top of the World Drive
Laguna Beach, CA 92651
949-715-7327 • www.basichealthpub.com

Library of Congress Cataloging-in-Publication Data
Schiller, David
    Aromatherapy for life empowerment : using essential oils to enhance
body, mind, spirit well-being / David Schiller and Carol Schiller.
        p. cm.
    Includes bibliographical references and index.
    ISBN 978-1-59120-285-1
    1. Aromatherapy. I. Schiller, Carol. II. Title.
    RM666.A68S3527   2011
    615'.3219—dc22
                                                    2010046354

Editor: Susan Davis
Typesetting/Book design: Gary A. Rosenberg
Cover design: Mike Stromberg
Front cover photograph: Jeffrey Schiller

Printed in the United States of America

10 9 8 7 6 5 4 3 2 1

Contents

Dedicated to you, our treasured reader.
May you gain the wisdom you seek
and your life be filled with
happiness, joy, and fulfillment.

Acknowledgments

We'd like to thank the following people and institutions:

Dr. Karl-Werner Quirin, Co-founder and President of Flavex, a high-quality producer of CO_2 extracts in Germany. The information in Chapter 1 on the CO_2 extraction process was provided courtesy of Dr. Quirin.

Stephen Pisano, Executive Vice President and Head of Purchasing of Organic Essential Oils at Citrus and Allied Essences, one of the most respected and high-integrity companies in the essential oil industry.

Mark Kerr, Managing Director of Tairawhiti Pharmaceuticals, a fine producer of high-quality manuka essential oil in New Zealand.

Norman Goldfind, Founder and Publisher of Basic Health Publications.

Gary Rosenberg, for his excellent design of this book.

Jeffrey Schiller, for providing the front cover photograph.

Cheryl Hirsch and Susan Davis, our editors.

Sharon Muir, for helping and encouraging many people to learn and become more knowledgeable about the magnificent uses of essential oils to improve their lives.

The public libraries, for their exceptional service. They are the greatest institutions for learning and are a vital asset to every community, providing enormous opportunities for those seeking to further their knowledge. Libraries serve as an invaluable resource of information, helping people become more informed and educated, which is vitally necessary in maintaining a free society.

We commend the following individuals and express our sincere appreciation for the helpful, caring, and unsurpassed service they provide at the Phoenix Public Library: Deputy Director of Branch Libraries Julaine Warner, Louis Howley, Greg Hills, Caren Lumley, Keith Cullers, Kathleen Birtciel, Judy De Bolt, Randle's Lunsford Jr., Debbie Fincher, Alex Latham, Rob Steele, Rita Martinez, Keith Feldt, Delphine Snowden, Jonathan Cole, Nancy Madden, Stephanie Martinez, Susan Clark, Karen Berner, Doris Foose, and Maritza Jerry.

The conscientious and diligent librarians and staff at the Glendale Public Library, especially: Joan Jensen, Stuart Levine, and Melanie Edens.

Nature's aromatic essences gently drifting through the air dispersing their aromas, seemingly appearing insignificant— yet having the unsurpassable ability to create and evoke powerful feelings, emotions, and memories that can last an entire lifetime.

—*David Schiller*

INTRODUCTION

Nature's Precious Essences

The magnificent fragrances and extraordinary beauty of nature's aromatic plants are unsurpassable. They enrich our life; bring us joy; embellish our surroundings; lift our spirit during illness; give us solace, comfort, and condolence in times of grieving; and heighten the festivity of every important occasion and celebration.

Aromatic plants have played an important role in the turn of events in history. Wars were fought to gain their possession, new lands were discovered in search for them, and cities that traded these valuable commodities became powerful centers of commerce. Some of the fragrant resins and oils derived from aromatic plants were in such great demand that they commanded prices comparable to, or even higher than, gold, silver, and precious jewels.

Today, we are fortunate that these precious oils are abundantly available for us to use. They offer simplistic solutions to sometimes difficult-to-solve problems, and they do it in a natural way.

There are 1,032 formulas provided in this book, offering a large variety of applications to choose from. You have the opportunity to select among the blends of essential oils that you have preference for and are most pleasing to your aromatic senses. Each formula can be made quickly, and is simple to use, even by a novice.

If you'd like to reduce your stress level, *Deep Breathing for Less Stress* (page 107) can assist in letting go of your tension. Getting a good night's sleep with *Sleep Peacefully* (page 114) may be the first formula you'll want to try.

Is there someone you'd like to get closer to, but have had difficulty communicating with on a deeper level? Perhaps the *Heart-to-Heart Talk* formulas (pages 74–77) can help. A good attitude increases the ability to get along better with people, so why not try the *Attitude Is Most Important* formulas (pages 30–32) to have better relationships with everyone you interact with?

Do you have a snorer in your house? Many marriages and families are put under duress when one person snores loudly, preventing the others from sleeping. Isn't it ironic that the snorer seems to always be the one who falls asleep first. *Stop Snoring!* (page 117) could be just what you and the snorer need.

More people are looking to minimize their exposure to synthetic chemicals in personal care products. One of your favorite formulas may be the *Freshen-Up Deodorants* (page 129) to help keep you feeling fresh all day, naturally. You can also make your own pure and natural face creams, body care creams, bath oils, bath salts, hair rinses, and more.

Who doesn't like a massage? The healing

touch from an aromatherapy massage is beneficial to our well-being. Choose from *Shoulder & Neck Release* (page 98), *Muscle & Joint Ease* (page 94), *Stress-Free Feet* (page 102), *Get Up & Go!* (page 92), *Back Renew* (page 89), and *Tummy Rub* (page 104). But that's not all. There's *Penetrating Chest Rub* (page 95), *Get Closer to Someone You Love* (page 91), *Seventh Heaven* (page 97), *Reward Yourself* (page 97), *Inner Peace* (page 92), and more.

The human mind is the greatest and most powerful creation on the face of the earth. Unfortunately, however, the mind is vastly underestimated and underutilized by many who do not recognize its phenomenal capability and potential to do good. Chapter 4, The Power of the Mind, offers a large variety of far-reaching formulas and exercises to encourage, inspire, empower, and greatly improve the quality of life within ourselves and in the lives of others. We were born with the potential for greatness and to have a meaningful life. Why settle for anything less? We have an obligation to live this greatness every day by the honorable intentions we manifest, the high–principled actions we take, and the harmonious relationships we develop with everyone around us.

Wouldn't you like to raise your vibration? The higher our vibration is, the better people, things, and events we attract to us. The *Higher Consciousness* (page 39) exercise practiced regularly can greatly help, and so can *Creating Good Karma* (page 32), *Intuition* (page 44), *Meditation* (page 50), *Practice Kindness* (page 83), *Be the Best You Can Be* (page 65), *Think Positive Thoughts* (page 61), *Wake Up to a Great Day!*

(page 86), *Make a Difference* (page 78), and *Reflection* (page 58). Dreams can give us important messages and intuitional insight. Perhaps you'll be eager to try one of the *Dream* formulas (pages 72–73).

Start the day off right by practicing the *Morning Affirmation* exercise (page 81), and carry out its meaningful purpose throughout the day. See the difference one simple affirmation makes; it only takes a few minutes to do! The *Mental Concentration* formulas (pages 52–54) can also be of great benefit. When you want to come up with creative ideas or any other situation that requires improved performance, these formulas will be there to help. And if you are active in body fitness and exercise, you'll really like the *Yoga & Exercise* application (page 119) to loosen up.

Do your family members get bitten up by mosquitoes? If so, the *Mosquito-Bandito Relief* (page 131) can come to the rescue and help soothe the area.

It doesn't take long for those who use the oils regularly to recognize their great value and respect their ability to perform effectively.

Practice the exercises and pursue a higher purpose, utilize your capabilities, raise your vibration, get greater fulfillment, become a good role model for others to follow, make a difference, create more happiness and joy within yourself, enrich your relationships, and get more out of life. Incorporate the aromatic oils every day and experience their positive impact. Feel empowered, treasure each moment, and be thankful for the extraordinary gift nature has given us—the precious essential oils.

CHAPTER 1

Aromatherapy Oils

In the past, when you've smelled an aroma, you've most likely only judged it from the standpoint of whether you liked it or not. Now you will learn to go far beyond that point by focusing primarily on how the oil affects you, rather than just liking or disliking it. Chances are you will find most of the oils to your liking. However, some of the oils that you may initially dislike may eventually become among your favorites after you've used them and experienced their wonderfully remarkable benefits.

ESSENTIAL OILS

Aromatherapy is the use of pure essential oils extracted from grasses, flower petals, seeds, fruit rinds, buds, resins, bark, wood, twigs, stems, leaves, roots, or rhizomes. Essential oils are responsible for the fragrance emitted by plants. These oils vary in color, are insoluble in water at room temperature, and have a watery consistency except for resins, some florals, as well as other essential oils like patchouli, sandalwood, and amyris, which tend to be heavier in viscosity.

The essential oil may be concentrated in a specific part of a plant or spread out in several areas. For example, the orange tree yields oil from its flower blossoms, leaves, twigs, and rind of the fruit. The clove tree contains oil in the buds, stems, and leaves. The whole plant of peppermint and lemongrass has oil, whereas essential oil is extracted only from the flowers of rose, jasmine, helichrysum, and ylang-ylang. See Table 1 for examples of the plant parts from which some essential oils are extracted.

Some essential oils are obtained from dried plant materials like allspice and clove buds; others are from fresh materials like neroli flowers, litsea cubeba berries, and the leaves of the eucalyptus citriodora tree. Some oils are extracted from ripe berries, such as juniper berry and litsea cubeba, and others are extracted from unripe berries, such as black pepper and allspice.

The quality and quantity of an essential oil produced from a plant depends on several factors: where the plant is grown (the altitude, moisture, climate), the condition of the soil, the season and time of day or night the plant material is harvested, and the extraction method used. The ylang-ylang tree bears flowers year-round, but the months in which the flowers contain the highest yield of oil are May and June. Rose petals are picked early in the morning before sunrise; jasmine flowers are picked at dusk before they are a day old.

Essential oils are highly volatile and evaporate when exposed to air. Carrier oils, also known as vegetal oils, are quite different than essential oils. They are extracted from nuts,

TABLE 1. EXAMPLES OF SPECIFIC PARTS OF PLANTS USED TO PRODUCE ESSENTIAL OILS	
ESSENTIAL OIL	PART OF PLANT THE OIL IS EXTRACTED FROM
Lemongrass, Palmarosa	Grass
Champaca Flower, Helichrysum, Jasmine, Neroli, Rose, Ylang-Ylang	Flowers
Chamomile, Clary Sage, Lavender, Marjoram	Flowering tops
Ginger, Spikenard, Vetiver	Roots
Amyris, Cabreuva, Cedarwood, Guaiacwood, Sandalwood	Wood chips
Cinnamon Leaf, Eucalyptus Citriodora, Eucalyptus Radiata, Patchouli, Ravensara, Sage	Leaves
Grapefruit, Lemon, Lime, Mandarin, Orange, Tangerine	Peel of the fruit
Copaiba	Resin
Allspice, Juniper Berry, Litsea Cubeba	Berries
Cardamom, Fennel	Seeds

seeds, fruits, and vegetables, and are made up of fatty acids, which give them a greasy texture. Carrier oils are used in aromatherapy to dilute the essential oils for massage applications, as well as for skin and hair care formulas. These oils protect the skin from possible irritation from the concentrated essential oils. Unlike essential oils, carrier oils are not as stable, have a shorter shelf life, and are not volatile.

We may not realize it, but practically everyone comes in contact with essential oils on many occasions each day. The oils are ingredients in toothpastes, chewing gum, candy, soft drinks, food flavorings, household products, cosmetics, perfumes, aftershave lotions, colognes, and skin, hair, and personal hygiene products. According to William Poundstone in the book *Big Secrets* (Harper, 1985), the proprietary formula for Coca-Cola includes the essential oils of nutmeg, cassia, lemon, orange, lime, neroli, lavender, and coriander.

METHODS OF EXTRACTION

The extraction process helps determine the purity of an oil. It is important to become knowledgeable about the different methods of extraction before purchasing essential and carrier oils.

Steam distillation. Steam from boiling water is used to release the essential oils from the plant material. The steam is then cooled and condensed into a liquid of water and essential oil. The oil separates and floats to the top, where where it is skimmed off. This extraction method is most extensively used and produces a good-quality essential oil.

Carbon dioxide (CO_2) extraction. CO_2 extraction is the most modern method available using high pressure and lower temperatures than steam distillation. There are two extracted types of oils using carbon dioxide (CO_2). One is called *Select*, the other is *Total*.

In CO_2 extraction, the plant material is placed into a chamber to which compressed CO_2 gas is released. The temperature is set to a range of 105–140°F (40–60°C). As the gas passes through the plant material, it draws out the components into solution.

The difference between the Select and the Total methods is in the amount of pressure used. This determines the density of the carbon dioxide gas and the ability of the gas to dissolve the plant material, as well as the viscosity of the oil. Select extracts are produced at 90–120 bar pressure, and the Total, 300–500 bar pressure.

When the process is completed, the pressure is lowered, and the extracted components precipitate out and are collected. The CO_2 gas is then recompressed and recycled to be used again, without leaving any residue in the extracted oil.

The Select oil contains components similar to the oils extracted through steam distillation. The Total method extracts a greater amount of the plant components. The oil is considered more identical to the plant material it's obtained from, containing more constituents than from the Select method. The Total oils tend to be thicker, and some are semisolid. This extract is comparable in components to the hexane solvent extracted oil.

An example is, when an extraction is done on the fennel plant, the Select extract consists of mainly essential oil, while the Total extract contains the essential oil together with the full amount of fatty oil (vegetal oil) that naturally occurs in the plant material.

Since the CO_2 process equipment is more costly, the extracted essential oils are more expensive than the steam distilled. However, CO_2 extracts have superior quality and composition.

Cold pressed citrus oils. Essential oils from citrus fruit require a different method of extraction. Citrus oils are extracted from the peel of the fruit, using a cold pressed method. The fruits are placed on a conveyor belt and then dropped into a cup with knives. As the cup closes, the knives puncture the fruit and remove the peel. The peel is then soaked in water and put through a centrifuge to separate out the essential oil.

Maceration. Plant material is soaked in hot fatty oil until its cells rupture and the oil absorbs the aromatic essence contained in the flowers.

Solvent extraction. The plant material is bathed in solvents, such as hexane and other toxic chemicals, which are used to extract the oil. Solvent extracted oils are less expensive to produce than the cold pressed, expeller pressed, steam distilled, and CO_2 extracted methods, and produce a higher yield. However, toxic residues remain in the oil, which makes this product undesirable for aromatherapy use. A high percentage of carrier/vegetal oils are extracted in this manner. Absolutes, such as jasmine, linden blossom, lotus, rose, and others are also produced with the use of solvents.

Cold pressed or expeller pressed extraction of carrier oils. Seeds, nuts, vegetables, and fruits are pressed without the use of high heat. These methods produce a quality oil.

Cold pressed oils are produced by a mechanical batch-pressing process in which heat-producing friction is minimized, so that temperatures remain below 120°F (49°C).

The expeller pressed method generates more heat to extract the oil, so in-line refrigerated cooling devices are added to the presses to keep the temperatures down to 185°F (85°C) during the pressing.

A large percentage of these oils are usually refined afterward using high heat and harsh chemicals. Therefore, it is important to check the product label on the container to ensure that the oil is unrefined so that it contains all the valuable nutrients.

Refining process of carrier oils. After the oil has been extracted from the plant material, it is usually put through a refining process that includes the following:

Degumming: Chlorophyll, vitamins, and minerals are removed from the oil.

Refining: An alkaline solution called lye is added to refine the oil.

Bleaching: Fuller's earth (a natural clay-like substance) is added as a bleaching agent and then filtered out to further remove nutritive substances; at this stage, the oil becomes clear.

Deodorizing: The oil is deodorized by steam distillation at high temperatures over 450°F (232° C) for 30 to 60 minutes.

Winterizing: The oil is then cooled and filtered. This process prevents the oil from becoming cloudy during cold temperatures.

The finished product is nutrient deficient, with only fatty acids remaining.

SYNTHETIC VERSUS NATURAL

Prior to the isolation of individual components of essential oils and the production of synthetic fragrances in the nineteenth century, the smell of an essence was representative of the plant material it originally came from. In today's synthetic fragrances, the true natural substances are mostly absent. The scent of a bouquet of flowers may not even contain one molecule of the essence of a real flower, or a food containing the flavoring of vanilla may smell and taste like vanilla, but yet it may not contain a drop of real vanilla.

Chemists are greatly skilled in their ability to cheaply produce synthetic versions of fragrances similar in scent to those of expensive essences. The purpose of their work is to create fragrant compounds to scent products and perfumes so that they are more appealing for purchase. However, these synthetic chemicals are no match when compared to the value of the natural essential oils.

Not only do synthetic compounds lack the beneficial properties of plants, but they can be irritating to the skin, respiratory system, and nervous system as well. Processing of these chemicals also pollutes the earth, water, and air. Essential oils, on the other hand, are much more than just a fragrance; they are the life force of the plants they are extracted from. These precious essences work on a much deeper level, affecting us not only on the physical but on the mental and spiritual level as well. They help balance the body, improve well-being, and put us into greater harmony with the natural world. They protect us with their antibacterial properties, reduce our stress, and give us comfort, reassurance, and pleasure.

HOW TO SELECT AND PURCHASE PURE OILS

It is unfortunate but a high percentage of essential oils commonly sold to the public are adulterated. This is done to increase profits without much concern for the consequences to the consumer. Some of the adulteration involves adding a cheaper oil to a more expensive oil in order to "stretch" it. See Table 2 for examples of common essential oil adulterations.

Many other more serious adulterations take place by adding fractionalized components, synthetic chemicals, and solvents, which contaminate the oils. This practice is common

TABLE 2. EXAMPLES OF ADULTERATION			
ESSENTIAL OIL	COMMONLY ADULTERATED WITH	ESSENTIAL OIL	COMMONLY ADULTERATED WITH
Allspice	Clove	Neroli	Orange, Petitgrain
Bergamot	Lime	Rose	Palmarosa
Cinnamon Bark	Cinnamon Leaf, Clove Leaf	Rosemary	Eucalyptus
Fennel (Sweet)	Fennel (Bitter)	Patchouli	Cedarwood, Copaiba, Gurjun Balsam
Geranium	Citronella, Palmarosa	Peppermint	Cornmint
Juniper Berry	Juniper wood and twigs	Sandalwood	Amyris, Cedarwood, Copaiba
Lavender	Lavandin	Ylang-Ylang	Cananga
Lemon	Orange		

knowledge in the essential oil industry and is referred to as "making a soup." Each time the oil changes hands, the possibility increases for the original oil to become more contaminated with adulterants.

Substantial variations exist in the prices that various essential oils sell for, as shown in Table 3. The factors that help determine price are:

1. The intensity of labor required to harvest the plant.

2. The extraction method used.

3. The yield of oil per plant.

4. The supply and demand for the particular plant material at a given time.

For example, in order to produce 1 pound of rose oil, over 4,000 pounds (1,800 kilograms) of roses must be picked and processed, whereas 1 pound ($1/_2$ kilogram) of lavender oil requires only about 250 pounds ($112 1/_2$ kilograms) of lavender flowers.

The highest-grade and most effective oils are produced from plants that are grown wild and away from polluted sources, or are cultivated by natural farming methods without the use of chemical pesticides, herbicides, or any other unnatural substances. It is important to select carrier oils that are cold or expeller pressed and unrefined, and essential oils that have been steam distilled, CO_2 extracted, or, in the case of citrus fruit oils, cold pressed.

TABLE 3. PRICES OF ESSENTIAL OILS VARY CONSIDERABLY FROM LEAST TO MORE EXPENSIVE	
Least Expensive	Anise, Cedarwood (Atlas), Cinnamon Leaf, Clove Bud, Copaiba, Eucalyptus Citriodora, Fennel (Sweet), Grapefruit, Lemon, Lime, Litsea Cubeba, Orange, Peppermint, Pine, Petitgrain, Rosemary, Sage, Spearmint, Tangerine
Moderately Expensive	Allspice Berry, Amyris, Basil (Sweet), Bergamot, Black Pepper, Clary Sage, Cumin, Cypress, Eucalyptus Radiata, Fir Needles, Geranium, Guaiacwood, Lavender, Mandarin, Marjoram (Spanish or Sweet), Patchouli, Ravensara Aromatica, Spruce, Thyme
More Expensive	Chamomile, Champaca Flower, Frankincense, Helichrysum, Hyssop Decumbens, Juniper Berry, Manuka (New Zealand Tea Tree), Myrtle, Neroli, Rose, Sandalwood, Spikenard, Vanilla, Ylang-Ylang

Retail oils are generally packaged in four different categories:

1. Individual pure essential oils with nothing added.

2. Carrier oils, found in a health food store, in the vegetable oil section.

3. Oil blends containing either a single essential oil mixed in a carrier oil, or several different essential oils mixed in a carrier oil.

4. Fragrance oils which are generally synthetic chemicals mixed together.

Investigating to find pure, high-quality oil is quite a learning experience, and it requires comparing the same oil of different brands with one another. Contacting the company and speaking with the appropriate person who oversees the purchasing of oils can help gain insight into the philosophy and integrity of the company.

CHAPTER 2

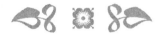

How to Use Aromatherapy

METHODS OF USE

Essential oils can be used in many ways. We can breathe them in while they are diffused or misted into the air, absorb them through our skin during a massage or application, and incorporate them as valuable aromatic ingredients to make an unlimited number of pure and natural products.

AIR DIFFUSION

The following are ways to diffuse essential oils into the air:

Aroma Lamps

There are a variety of beautiful and decorative aroma lamps that can be used in the home or at the office.

To Use: Fill the small container on top of the aroma lamp with water and add the essential oils. Depending on the type of aroma lamp you have, light the candle or turn on the light bulb. As the water heats, the fragrance of the oil diffuses into the air.

Diffusers

Diffusers disperse a mist of essential-oil micro - particles, which create an aromatic atmosphere for the indoors. There are different types of dif-

fusers on the market. You can choose a smaller or larger unit, depending on the size of the area to be fragranced.

The formulas given in Chapters 5 and 8 for diffuser use are in percentages rather than drops because of the different types of units available. The essential oils are either (1) added to a pad and warmed by an electrical heating element that diffuses the aroma into the air; or (2) placed into a small glass bottle and propelled with a gentle air current into a nebulizer and vaporized into the air.

BATHS

Soaking in warm water scented with essential oils can be so pleasurable that once you experience an aromatic bath, plain water baths will become a thing of the past.

To prepare: Select one of the bath oil formulas in Chapter 8. Close the bathroom door and window(s) to keep the warm steam of the bathwater and essential oil vapors from escaping out of the room. Then fill the bathtub with water as warm as you like and turn on soft music. Mix the essential oils with the carrier oil. To use: Pour the formula into the bathwater. Swirl the water to distribute the oils evenly throughout the tub and enter the bath immediately. Enjoy the wonderful aromas!

CREAMS

Creams help nourish, moisturize, and assist in bringing about soft and beautiful-looking skin. They apply easily and have a smooth texture. Natural unrefined cocoa butter and unrefined shea butter are used in the cream formulas provided in Chapter 8.

To prepare: Place the indicated amount of the vegetable butter into a wide-mouthed glass jar, put the jar into a small pot of water, and heat on a low temperature. When the butter melts, add the carrier oil, mix well, and remove from the heat. As the mixture cools, add the essential oils, stir well, and tightly cap the jar. To use: Wait until the cream cools completely and becomes creamy in texture before using. Place a label on the jar and store in a dark, cool place.

INHALERS

Inhalers are convenient to use and provide quick results.

To prepare: Combine the essential oils in a small $1/4$ ounce (7.5 ml) or $1/2$ ounce (15 ml) glass bottle with a wide opening. Tighten the cap and gently shake to mix the oils. Place a label on the bottle and store in a dark, cool place. To use: Relax in a comfortable chair, open the bottle, and slowly inhale the vapors 15 to 20 times. Breathe deeply. Cap the bottle immediately after use and store for the next time.

Over time the inhaler may lose its potency as the vapors become faint. At that point, there is no need to discard the formula. Instead, reuse the oils by combining them in a fine-mist glass spray bottle with purified water and add fresh essential oils to use as a mist spray (see Mist Sprays on page 11).

MASSAGE

One of the most satisfying pleasures in life is receiving an aromatherapy massage in a relaxed, peaceful ambience with a comfortable temperature setting and soft music playing in the background. Taking time out to experience this wonderful, nurturing form of touch in a tranquil environment can be helpful to improve health and overall well-being. Chapter 6 is devoted to massage formulas.

For best results when giving a massage, please follow these guidelines:

- Wear comfortable clothing.
- Fingernails should be short.
- Use a massage table or place a firm cushion on the floor to do the massage on.
- Be in a calm and positive state of mind, since tension can easily be transferred to the receiver during the massage.
- A spray mist can be used prior to the receiver coming into the room.
- Choose the appropriate massage formula, and place all oils nearby to avoid searching for them during the massage.
- Wash hands with warm water before and after giving the massage.
- Warm the carrier oil by placing the small container in warm water. Pour an ample amount into the palm of your hand, rub hands together, and then apply the oil on the receiver's skin.
- After the massage, use arrowroot powder or cornstarch to dry off any remaining oil on the skin.

MIST SPRAYS

A convenient and effective way to disperse aromatic vapors in the air is through the use of a mist spray. As the aromas mature in the bottle, the fragrance improves.

To prepare: Fill a fine-mist spray glass bottle with purified water, add the essential oils, and tightly cap the bottle. Label and store in a dark, cool place. To use: Shake the bottle well. Sit comfortably in a chair. Position the sprayer a few inches over the head so that the mist falls in front of the face. Close the eyes and spray approximately ten or more times. Stop after every two to three sprays and inhale deeply.

SELF-APPLICATION

This method is used when there isn't another person available to give a massage. The oils should be rubbed into the skin until they are fully absorbed. When done, apply and rub a small amount of arrowroot powder or cornstarch onto the area to remove any remaining oil from the skin.

COMMON MISTAKES

In order to obtain maximum results, it is important to avoid these commonly made mistakes:

- Not fully massaging the formulas into the skin. The oils should be massaged in for at least 30 minutes.

- Wiping off the oil that remains on the skin after a massage or self-application with a tissue or towel. Instead, rub in arrowroot powder or cornstarch to dry off the remaining oil from the skin.

- Not inhaling deeply enough the vapors from the inhaler and mist spray formulas. By not inhaling deeply, hardly any vapors enter the breathing passages.

- Not misting the mist sprays properly. It is important that the mist falls in front of the face with eyes closed.

- Using stimulating essential oils before bedtime.

- Using sleep-inducing essential oils during the daytime.

- Carelessly applying essential oils near the eyes and other sensitive areas of the body. Irritation can result, causing discomfort.

- Leaving bottles of oils exposed to direct light and not using dark-colored glass bottles to store oils in. The effectiveness of the oils is reduced when they are improperly stored.

HELPFUL MEASUREMENTS				
Liquid Measurements	1 teaspoon	0.16 fluid ounce	5 milliliters	4.73 grams
	2 teaspoons	0.33 fluid ounce	10 milliliters	9.75 grams
	3 teaspoons (1 tablespoon)	0.5 fluid ounce	15 milliliters	14.70 grams
	6 teaspoons (2 tablespoons)	1 fluid ounce	30 milliliters	29.50 grams
	8 teaspoons (2 tablespoons + 2 teaspoons)	1.35 fluid ounces	40 milliliters	39.90 grams
Dry Measurements	4 tablespoons ($^1/_4$ cup)	2 ounces	60 milliliters	56.70 grams
	8 tablespoons ($^1/_2$ cup)	4 ounces	120 milliliters	113.40 grams
	16 tablespoons (1 cup)	8 ounces	240 milliliters	225.00 grams

SAFETY, STORAGE, AND HANDLING OF OILS

Please follow these guidelines for the safe and proper use of the essential oils:

- Essential oils are highly concentrated substances. To prevent the possibility of skin irritation, always dilute essential oils in a carrier oil, such as almond (sweet), hazelnut, or sesame oil, before applying on the skin. Should any irritation occur as a result of the essential oils, apply additional carrier oil to the area and increase the amount of carrier oil in the formula. If irritation persists, apply cornstarch and discontinue use of the formula.

- If a person has sensitive skin, discretion should be used for the application and massage formulas: Apply additional carrier oil to the skin area, increase the amount of carrier oil in the formula, reduce the number of essential oil drops in the formula, choose blends with oils that are gentle on the skin, or use non-topical methods such as mist sprays and inhalers instead. There are people with extremely sensitive skin who cannot tolerate essential oils without experiencing skin irritation. If this is the case, discontinue use.

- If someone is highly allergic, use this simple and easy test to determine if there is any ensitivity to a specific oil: Rub a drop of carrier oil on the upper chest area. In twelve hours, check the skin for redness or any other reaction. If the skin is clear, place one drop of an essential oil in twenty drops of the same carrier oil that was tested to be safe and again rub the mixture on the upper chest area. If no skin reaction occurs after twelve hours, both the carrier oil and the essential oil should be fine to use.

- Be careful not to get the oils or their vapors in the eyes. If this occurs, flush with cool water.

- As a precaution, many essential oils aren't used during pregnancy due to the stimulating effect they can have on the urinary system and uterus. Even certain common foods, spices, and vegetable oils, such as celery, carrots, parsley, basil, bay leaves, marjoram, as well as safflower oil, can stimulate uterine contractions. Small amounts of two or three drops at one time of the following essential oils are said to be safe during pregnancy: bergamot, coriander, cypress, frankincense, geranium, ginger, grapefruit, lavender, lemon, lime, mandarin, neroli, orange, patchouli, petitgrain, sandalwood, spearmint, tangerine, ylang-ylang. The carrier oil of sesame can be used in normal quantities. The greatest risk to pregnant women is using essential oils that are adulterated with chemical solvents. Purity is of the utmost importance.

- Nursing mothers should use extra care in the selection of essential oils, especially for skin application, since the effects of the oils are transferred to the infant.

- Do not consume alcohol, except for a small glass of wine with a meal, in the time period when using essential oils.

- Do not use essential oils while on medication as the oils might interfere with the medicine.

- Avoid sunbathing, tanning booths, or using the sauna/steam room for at least four hours after using citrus and other essential oils that can irritate the skin. Phototoxic oils can cause the skin to burn when exposed to sunlight. See precautions in the Essential Oil Profiles, Chapter 10.

• When spilled on furniture, many essential oils will remove the finish; therefore, be careful when handling the bottles.

• Light and oxygen cause carrier and essential oils to deteriorate rapidly. Refrigeration does not prevent spoilage but diminishes the speed at which it occurs; therefore, oils should be stored in amber-colored glass bottles in a dark, cool place.

• Always use a glass dropper when measuring drops of essential oil.

• Keep all bottles tightly closed to prevent the oils from evaporating and oxidizing.

• After mixing carrier and essential oils together, use as soon as possible or within six months to avoid the possibility of spoilage.

• Always store essential oils out of sight and reach of children.

• Clearly label all bottles and jars that contain blends.

CHAPTER 3

❧ ❀ ❧

Experiencing Aromatherapy

Many people become greatly intrigued after smelling the aromas of the essential oils, but there's so much more to be experienced. When used regularly, the oils can affect us on our deepest levels—lifting the spirit, awakening the senses, stirring the emotions, touching the heart, and enlivening every part of our being. Some oils work instantly; others are more subtle and take longer. Some will warm you on a cold winter day, while others will cool you in the heat of the summer. The energizing oils are best used early in the day, while the relaxants are best before bedtime. Some of the aromas are instantly liked; others take time to get used to. In due time with experience, you will be able to select the oils that are right for each occasion.

You may start to notice some very interesting occurrences taking place as you do the following Essential Oil Analysis exercise. Certain aromas may trigger memories you hadn't thought of in a while—some enjoyable, others perhaps you need to deal with. Some people may discover they are so wound up with stress that as they start to calm down, they may feel uneasy and actually resist becoming relaxed. Their body is subconsciously accustomed to this stressful condition that it keeps resisting change for the better. If this is the case, give yourself permission to release your stress and try one of the *Soothe Nervous Tension* formulas in Chapter 6 or *Peace & Calm* in Chapter 7. The more you practice letting go, the easier it will become.

Aromatherapy encourages us to gain greater understanding of how scents affect us. Explore, learn, discover, involve yourself; get acquainted with many of the scents you are currently unfamiliar with. Allow your senses to be taken on a fascinating journey and be open to enjoying more of the simple pleasures in life. Observe, pay close attention to your feelings, moods, and passing thoughts, and don't overlook the vital importance of the messages the scents bring.

ESSENTIAL OIL ANALYSIS EXERCISE

To understand and fully appreciate how each individual essential oil affects you, set up the following items and do the exercise.

Items Needed

- Carrier oil
- Essential oils
- Glass droppers
- Arrowroot powder or cornstarch
- A pen or pencil
- Make a copy of the Essential Oil Analysis Form for Mental, Mood, and Emotional

Changes and the Essential Oil Analysis Form for Physical Changes at the end of this chapter.

Instructions

1. Find a peaceful and comfortable room where you can relax. Make sure you will not be disturbed by the telephone, doorbell, people entering the room, or noisy pets.

2. Play soft music (optional) to help create a relaxing mood.

3. Place the items necessary for this exercise where you will be sitting.

4. Add a feeling of tranquility to the room by adjusting the lighting.

5. Relax in a comfortable chair or on a cushion on the floor.

6. Apply approximately 20 drops of carrier oil on your wrist and forearm. The carrier oil should coat the entire skin area. Gently rub both wrists and forearms together to distribute the oil evenly.

7. Select an essential oil and apply one drop over the carrier oil on one of your wrists and gently rub the oil into the skin. Close your eyes and bring your wrists up toward your nose without touching your face or nostrils. Slowly inhale the vapors. Sit quietly for 5 to 10 minutes; clear your mind, relax your body, and focus on the benefits of the oil according to the categories listed on the worksheets. The more you relax the easier it will be to experience the effects of the essential oil.

8. Fill out both Essential Oil Analysis Forms on pages 17 and 18.

9. To dull the scent on the skin from one oil to another, rub a small amount of arrowroot powder or cornstarch over the area where the previous essential oil was applied. To evaluate the next essential oil, repeat instructions 6 and 7.

Words to Describe Scents

Balsamic	Irritating	Pungent
Bitter	Lemony	Refreshing
Camphoraceous	Minty	Salty
Citrusy	Musky	Smokey
Earthy	Musty	Spicy
Floral	Orangy	Sweet
Fruity	Penetrating	Vaporous
Herbaceous	Piercing	Woody

ESSENTIAL OIL ANALYSIS FORM
FOR MENTAL, MOOD, & EMOTIONAL CHANGES*

ESSENTIAL OIL	CHANGES*	MEMORIES EVOKED	CONCLUSION
1.			
2.			
3.			
4.			
5.			
6.			
7.			
8.			
9.			
10.			

MENTAL, MOOD, & EMOTIONAL CHANGES

A = Aphrodisiac	IA = Increases Awareness	RS = Reduces Stress
AL = Alert, Mentally	IC = Increases Confidence	RT = Restless
C = Comforting	IN = Invigorating	RV = Reviving
D = Dulls the Mind	IT = Increases Tension/Stress	SE = Serene
E = Euphoric	MC = Mental Clarity	SO = Soothing
EX = Excited	MU = Mood Uplifting	ST = Still
H = Happy	Q = Quiet	STM = Stimulating
I = Irritated Mood	RJ = Rejuvenating	

* Please make a copy of this sheet and fill it out.

ESSENTIAL OIL ANALYSIS FORM FOR PHYSICAL CHANGES*

ESSENTIAL OIL	PREFERENCE	BODY AREA AFFECTED	CHANGES	BODY TEMP.	WEIGHT SENSATION	COMMENTS
1.						
2.						
3.						
4.						
5.						
6.						
7.						
8.						
9.						
10.						

PREFERENCE	BODY AREA AFFECTED	CHANGES	BODY TEMPERATURE	WEIGHT SENSATION
L = Like	AB = Abdomen	BE = Breathing Easier	C = Cooling	L = Light Body Feeling
D = Dislike	AR = Arms	C = Calming	W = Warming	H = Heavy Body Feeling
I = Indifferent	B = Back	E = Energizing	NC = No Change	NC = No Change
	C = Chest	IT = Increased Tension		
	H = Head	ML = Muscle Loosener		
	L = Legs	P = Pain Relief		
	N = Neck	TR = Tension Relief		
	S = Spine			

* Please make a copy of this sheet and fill it out.

CHAPTER 4

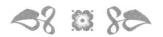

The Power of the Mind

The incredible human brain is the most complex structure of living cells known in the universe. The brain is extraordinary and remarkable, but yet unparalleled as the most underutilized part of the body according to its capability and potential. It weighs approximately three pounds (1.35 kilograms), consumes about 20 percent of the body's oxygen intake, and contains up to 100 billion neurons (brain cells) and a greater number of glial cells that nourish and service the neurons. Unlike other brains in the animal kingdom, the human brain possesses the ability of a higher consciousness to think logically, reason, and plan; great creative imagination to envision what is not yet in existence; and the capability to take action to carry out a vision until it becomes reality.

The brain can provide a person with the ability to generate extraordinary thoughts and ideas to build magnificent structures, machinery, equipment, and tools; devise clever ways to overcome obstacles to make life easier; trigger the emotions of love, compassion, and warmth; and provide care and comfort for the sick and needy. It also can create peace, harmony, accord, healing, enlightenment, cooperation, and good will. On the other hand, the brain can produce conflict, deception, betrayal, discord, strife, belligerency, and hostility. And can help develop and make the most disastrous weapons of war,

which, when used, bring great pain, suffering, and annihilation to large numbers of people and other living things. Each one of us chooses the purposes for which we want to use our brain. To be productive and constructive, or destructive—the choice is ours to make.

THE POWER OF OUR THOUGHTS

The mind can only focus on one thought at a time. Everything begins with a single thought. One thought can change the temperature in your body, create stress and tension, make you sad, angry, nervous, and jittery, or happy, elated, ecstatic, enthusiastic, appreciative, calm, and peaceful. A thought can affect your metabolic functions, digestion, breathing, pulse rate, and blood pressure. One thought can also trigger emotions and influence your attitude and the decisions you make. One thought can initiate acts to start a conflict, and one thought in the mind of caring people can help seek solutions to make peace.

Thoughts create our physical reality. Negative thoughts activate the body into a fight-or-flight mode. In this state, all the body's resources are put on alert and mobilized for immediate action, while other bodily functions, such as digestion, assimilation, blood cell production, and healing are put on hold.

The emergency chemicals that are produced in this reaction, if they are unused, eventually begin breaking down into toxic substances. The muscles stay tense, especially around the neck, shoulders, chest, and abdomen. Positive thoughts bring about a favorable condition for the functions of the body to thrive and a more conducive environment for healing and a state of well-being to occur.

Higher Consciousness

Every living being is a body of energy that emits frequencies. The frequency produced attracts people, things, and events to us whose resonance is in sync with the same range of vibration as ours.

Living in higher consciousness is the highest form of existence. It is the level of striving to attain the highest reward of inner satisfaction that life has to offer. A person cannot comprehend what the good feeling of this state is unless they live in it. The greater the number of individuals who have higher levels of consciousness, the greater the possibility for people to get along with one another and peace to take place between nations.

The physical and spiritual worlds differ greatly. In the physical realm, if we work hard and smart, we may be rewarded by becoming successful, receiving greater compensation, and having the capability to acquire more material possessions. This process is easily visible. Wealth can be measured in terms of money and acquisition. In the spiritual realm, when we do the right thing, learn our lessons, take on a healthy attitude, and develop greater levels of honesty, compassion, kindness, and forgiveness, it works on the inside to feed and nourish the needs of our soul. However, the results are subtle, and our reward is felt on the inside and on the outside. This kind of wealth cannot be measured in the physical realm, but this is who we really are.

If you want to live in a better world, show a good example by the way you conduct yourself. Whatever wrongs you see taking place, counteract them by your virtuous actions. If you see unfairness, be fair; if you see cruelty, be kind; if you see hatred, be loving; if you see disrespect, be respectful; if you see dishonesty, be honest; if you see conflict, be peaceful; if you see ungratefulness, be grateful; if you see indifference to suffering, be compassionate; if you see others who are uncaring, be caring; if you see hurt and loss, be comforting; if you see people being dishonorable, be honorable; if you see untruthfulness, speak the truth; if you hear idle talk, rumors, and gossip, be smart and don't engage; and if you see people who are in darkness, be the light.

The worst excuse a person can have for doing wrong is: "I did it because everyone else was doing it." Whether it is a child misbehaving with friends in school, a person who is part of a lynch mob, or a soldier involved in committing genocide, just because the crowd does it, doesn't mean it is right. Use your own thinking ability and think for yourself.

Here are twenty-two virtues to attain higher consciousness. By practicing these virtues daily, we can greatly improve the meaning of our life and the lives of those around us.

1. Have self-discipline: Discipline is inner strength and is necessary for self-mastery.

2. Be honest: Honesty is the foundation of goodness. The more honest we are, the better we feel about ourselves. Honesty is required to build the other virtues on.

3. Be truthful: Live the truth and you will feel better about yourself.

4. Be grateful: Gratefulness is an important

part of living a meaningful life and having inner happiness.

5. Have integrity: High integrity earns respect. Maintain the highest standards and ethical values; take the high road.

6. Take action: Get involved by doing. Don't put things off.

7. Be trustworthy: Earn people's trust by acting in a responsible way.

8. Keep your word: Practice what you preach; do as you say. If you give your word, follow through in a timely manner.

9. Be kind: Make sure every day to practice acts of kindness. When you do a kind act, do it out of goodness in your heart. Don't expect anything back in return.

10. Take control of yourself: You are a sacred being. Choose to live a healthy lifestyle and take the best care of yourself that you can.

11. Don't blame others: If you blame others you deny yourself the opportunity to learn and grow. Take responsibility for your actions and inactions, and don't feel sorry for yourself.

12. Be forgiving: When you forgive another person, it helps you to free yourself from a heavy burden. You don't have to forget, but forgive the wrongdoing and let it go.

13. Be a peacemaker: Do your best to live in peace with the people around you.

14. Have persistence: Pay attention to your conscience. If you know you are doing the right thing, keep doing it.

15. Connect with the higher source: The power that created us wants the best for each of us.

16. Be the best you can be: Why would anyone choose to live a life being less than his or her potential? Put the time and effort into developing yourself as a person, as well as your skills and talents.

17. Think for yourself: Keep your own individuality and use your own thinking ability. Look into and question things; do your own research. This will help you make better decisions.

18. Spend time in a quiet place: Set aside important time to reflect and be open to receive ideas about what you can do to handle your life challenges more successfully.

19. Respect life: Everything is here for a purpose. Treat the life of other beings with respect.

20. Right your wrongs: An uneasy conscience can be the result of the wrongs we've done in the past and can cause agonizing inner turmoil and discomfort. Be responsible; make amends and restitution to those you have wronged, and correct your ways.

21. Have compassion: Be sensitive to the distress of other beings. Raise the level of goodness in your heart.

22. Simplify your life: Find ways to simplify your life one step at a time. Things become less difficult when you practice simplicity.

Make a copy of these twenty-two virtues and rate yourself from 1 to 5 for each one. When you've completed this exercise, write down on a separate sheet of paper the virtues you need to improve on, and start working on them. Use the Higher Consciousness formulas on pages 39–41.

Intuition

Everyone has a degree of intuition, though it is more developed and used by some individuals than others. Intuition is a strong feeling of wisdom, an inner voice providing us with valuable information and insight. Its role is vital; yet the messages are frequently ignored by those who do not understand or trust their inner voice.

Dreams have been recognized as a source of intuitional insight. In David Ryback's book *Dreams That Come True* (Doubleday, 1988), Rybeck writes about a mother who had a dream that she was in a funeral home and all her son's friends were coming to her to express their condolences because they said her son was killed in an auto accident. Also present were friends and relatives who had previously passed on. They told her this was only a warning of what would happen if her son wasn't careful.

The next day, the mother told her son about the dream and warned him to be careful driving. A few weeks later, the son was driving 70 to 80 miles an hour when he suddenly thought about the message his mother had given him. He slowed down immediately, and right after, one of the car's tires blew out. He was able to control the car and pull over safely to the side of the road. Had he not slowed down, the vehicle could have gone out of control and caused severe injuries or possibly death.

In one of our aromatherapy classes, a young lady, about twenty years old, was planning to get married in a few months. For her homework assignment, she used a dream formula and during the night had a dream that her fiancé was looking for her with the intention to seriously harm her. She hid underneath her bed hoping he would not find her. When she awoke, she shrugged off what she had dreamt and considered it to be just a bad dream. When she came to the next class, she presented the details of the dream. She was then asked if her fiancé had previously shown any tendencies toward violent behavior and if she had any reservations about getting married. She replied that he was a wonderful person and that she was looking forward to the wedding. Two years later, she divorced her husband on the grounds of physical abuse and the possible endangerment of her life. He had threatened to kill her if she ever left him.

Another student had a dream that she came early to a party and read the list of all the guests who were invited. Two days after the dream, she returned home from work not knowing that her mother had arranged a surprise party for her and invited friends and former classmates she knew from many years ago. The people who were at the party were the same people whose names appeared on the guest list in her dream. She was shocked!

As these examples prove, dreams can offer enormously useful insights. While intuition emanates from the right side of the brain, it is best to combine it for decision making with the left side of the brain where logic and reasoning predominate. (Dream formulas are on pages 72–73.)

Karma

Karma is the universal law of cause and effect. You reap what you sow; every action causes an equal reaction. Thoughts, words, and actions are the cause, and the experiences they trigger are the effect. Every action leaves an imprint, and the imprint eventually gives rise to its own individual effect.

Karma is a power that exerts a force to cause a person to change for the better. Since people are resistant to change, they view the pressure to change as negative. Numerous chances are given over time, but if the improvement does not take place, the force increases.

The occurrence of so much pain and suffering inflicted by people on one another all over the world clearly shows they don't realize, believe, or fully accept the extent to which the law of karma works. The reason they may think this way is because karmic payback doesn't usually occur instantly; therefore, they are unable to make the direct connection of the cause and the effect.

Life on earth is our school, and we are given many tests. The universe teaches a person who did a wrongdoing what it feels like to be the recipient of the act. We keep getting tested on an ongoing basis to measure the progress we've made. For example, a person who has stopped drinking alcohol will be invited to an event where many are drinking to see if he has developed enough discipline to abstain. A married man with children is attracted to a woman coworker and is tempted to have a relationship with her. Both are being tested to see if they will jeopardize breaking up a marriage and decimating a family just to fill their own selfish desires. A woman finds a wallet, giving her an opportunity to prove her honesty by returning the wallet and its full contents to the rightful owner.

Every time we pass a test, we feel better about ourselves and create better karma.

Bad karma can even be earned by a person engaging in addictions and self-destructive behavior. When people do harm to themselves, not only do they cause their own suffering, which is a violation, but they also cause hurt on others they are close to, which is another violation. For example, when a person who smokes cigarettes comes down with cancer, just think how affected his or her spouse, children, family, and friends are from the illness and suffering the person goes through.

Parents can earn karma by the way they interact with their children. To overprotect a child and stifle his or her growth and development is very negative, while a parent who encourages learning, self-development, honesty, and high moral character values earns good karma.

Some people may think that bad karma leads to a shortened life, but that doesn't seem to be true. People with accumulated bad karma can live long lives. The reason for this may be to give them more time to make good for the wrongs they have done.

It is important to start creating good karma from this moment on to offset and correct some of the unfair and unjust acts we've committed in the past. Meritorious actions can turn our karma around to the positive side.

Motives for Our Actions

Two people can perform the same act, yet each person can have a different motive for doing so. For example, one woman helps a sick relative because she anticipates receiving a large inheritance in reward for her actions. Another woman helps a sick relative out of compassion and caring for a human being and seeks no reward in return. It is important to examine our motives of why we do things and what we expect in return.

Reflection

When our life on earth is through, what will have mattered are the principles we stood for, what we did for the ones we loved, the goodness and kindness we imparted to those around us, the beauty and treasures we recognized and appreciated that others took for granted, the example we set by the way we lived, the people's hearts we touched, and the fond memories we gave to those we knew.

Our thoughts, hopes, and actions of today play a key role in contributing to the shape of our world of tomorrow. It is vital to probe ourselves periodically to assess and evaluate our general purpose and direction in life. Just as a captain navigates a ship, we must know our position and steer our course toward our desired destination.

Introspection

Look inside, examining thoughts, feelings, and reasoning for self-observation. Many of us are so absorbed in our work and daily affairs that we seldom take the time to examine our inner thoughts and feelings or evaluate the extent to which we honor our promises, commitments, and responsibilities to relatives, business associates, friends, acquaintances, and others in our life.

Improvement

The price to pay to improve and become a better person is much less costly than the price to pay to be anything less than the best we can be. We come here with a purpose for our life. We are given talents and gifts that we need to develop and refine.

Every day we have the opportunity to acquire additional knowledge, think of new ideas, improve ourselves, and make life more meaningful. Perhaps the greatest chance we have to improve, which few people take advantage of, is giving consideration when we are offered constructive criticism. Many people find it difficult to accept; they get upset and defensive. Everyone seems to enjoy being complimented, but hardly anyone is receptive to criticism.

People who care about us point out key observations to try to help us. It takes a special, caring person who has the courage to do so, sometimes at the risk of offending someone and losing a friendship. Be grateful and appreciative; accept the criticism in a positive way, just as you would like others to take criticism that you give

them. Reflect on how this valuable advice can help you improve. This course of contemplation can prove to be an invaluable tool as you progress along the path of life.

Motivation

Motivation drives a person to do things. Every action we take can be attributed to motivation. We take actions that we perceive will bring us pleasure and satisfaction, and we back away from what we perceive as fearful and painful.

Motivation is a driving force that, in order to be genuine and lasting, must come from within the person. If someone requires a pep talk, motivation from attending a seminar or reading a book, it is a good way to get started, but that will only yield temporary results. Motivation that comes from the outside can only magnify the motivation that already exists inside. It cannot create motivation over the long term where none exists internally.

When motivation originates from the inside, it goes hand and hand with conviction, enthusiasm, strength, and perseverance, which are valuable characteristics in the achievement of success.

Self-motivation makes a person excel. The most powerful tool is a motivated human being.

Loving Yourself

Life is very fragile, especially at the very beginning. Different factors are important for proper development and well-being.

Newborn animals rely on their mother's touch; otherwise, they will die within the first few hours after birth.

Throughout the nineteenth century, large numbers of children who were raised in orphanages and didn't receive touch died from a disease called "wasting away." As late as the 1920s, the death rate for infants under one year of age in orphanages throughout the United States was over 60 percent.

It is very unfortunate to see high numbers of children grow up without bonding with their parents and feeling unloved, unwanted, and uncared for. It is unfortunate this carries through to other relationships over a person's lifetime, causing much pain and suffering. Many people engage in self-destructive behavior: overeating, smoking, or drinking excessive quantities of alcohol. This may be a result of negative childhood conditioning or could have been acquired over the years of dealing with a lifestyle that was overly stressful and frustrating. Free yourself by relinquishing habits that are harmful, replacing them with activities and behavior that give you great joy and satisfaction and that help you feel good about yourself.

If we don't love ourselves, who can we love? And who can we expect to love us? Good relationships are created not only by finding the right person, but also by first being the right person.

We must learn to love ourselves, starting right now—no matter how terrible we've felt about past actions and our life situation. Let all that go. Each day life begins anew.

Think of a person whom you had great love

Loving Yourself Affirmation

I am a valuable, precious, unique, and special being of the light.

I honor and treasure the creation of my existence. I celebrate who I am; I wouldn't change with anyone else in the world.

I open myself up to receive the wondrous miracles and blessings from the higher power.

I embrace my inner knowing and wisdom. My higher self guides and encourages me to be kind and caring to myself.

I am worthy of love. I know that the love has to come from deep within my inner self.

I am my own best friend, and the greatest possession I have.

The love I have within is my greatest healer.

I enjoy my own company. I know I'll be living with myself for the rest of my life. I take positive actions and derive positive feelings. I find peace within by living it.

I grow and improve more each day in self-discipline, self-mastery, self-reliance, and self-caring.

I choose higher thoughts no matter what the challenges are.

I develop and maintain loving relationships and impart kind words to uplift and inspire all who I come in contact with.

Today is a new beginning, alive, fresh with enormous enthusiasm, great purpose and special meaning.

I am now fully committed to start anew, letting go of the past and taking full responsibility for giving myself the best life I possibly can.

for. Think of how joyous and wonderful you felt being around this person. Now, how about feeling the same love for yourself?

Forgiveness

It is unfortunate that we are sometimes wronged, but to carry the feeling of unforgiveness around makes it worse. Forgiveness is necessary for healing to take place. It is disconnecting from the hurt we have accumulated. We need to let go and overcome anger, resentment, animosity, and hostility against the person or persons who we feel have hurt us. To seek revenge, to get even, or to wish ill will on another person, brings negative karma. We can make a choice to forgive.

When a person gets upset and angry, many parts of the body become adversely affected. The adrenal glands release adrenaline and the body goes into a fight-or-flight survival mode. As a result, the body becomes tight, the heart rate quickens, blood pressure rises, breathing becomes faster, and digestion turns off. If the anger is held onto by the person, it turns into resentment, continuing the same process, but on a more subtle, less drastic level than when the anger first took place. As the condition continues, circulation becomes impeded, especially in certain areas of the body. This creates an unhealthy state, and is why the process of forgiveness is so necessary to let go and rid the body of the enormous burden. This is an important step to take to help encourage the restoration of good health.

Appreciation

In this fast-paced lifestyle we rush through our lives, on many occasions failing to acknowledge inwardly and outwardly the people and things we have to be thankful for. Take time to feel appreciative for all you have. Give thanks for having food, shelter, clothing, friends, family, and even a pet. One cannot experience the joy of true happiness while taking the necessities of life for granted.

Meditation

Meditation relaxes the metabolism to a lower point than sleep, as the body gains a deep, concentrated level of rest. The rate of breathing and the amount of oxygen intake decreases and so does the blood pressure and heartbeat rate.

Meditation is a quieting of the conscious mind. The stillness of this state allows deeper levels of relaxation and peacefulness to be attained. It enables a greater ability to focus and allows thoughts to develop. This is a state in which the mind does not engage in judgment or analysis. There is awareness of all thoughts that arise, but these thoughts are allowed to pass by without being analyzed. People who practice meditation regularly respond to stressful situations more effectively and thus decrease stress levels and anxiety dramatically.

The benefits of meditation are cumulative and offer profound improvement to physical and emotional health. It is important to practice these exercises regularly to achieve best results.

Visualization

Visualization is an innate process of using our thoughts and imagination to create a picture in our mind of a goal we are seeking to accomplish. We practice mental imagery regularly on many occasions without realizing it. Everything we do in life originates in the mind as a thought or a vision. We are visualizing when we imagine ourselves living in a new house or visiting a new country. Often our ideas progressively develop into a tangible goal. This process is the vital doorway that enables us to see and plan for what we want in life.

When wanting to achieve a specific goal, it is important first to make sure it is realistic and attainable. Then support your goal with an outline of a plan of action and the time frame in which you would like to see it come to fruition. Remember: The major factor that will determine your success hinges upon the strength of your desire to achieve—your determination and your purpose for doing it.

GUIDELINES TO PREPARE FOR RELAXATION

Many of the formulas in this chapter require doing the relaxation exercise.

- Find a peaceful and comfortable place to relax.
- Make sure you will not be disturbed by the telephone, doorbell, people entering the room, or noisy pets.
- The room temperature should be warm.

- Soft music in the background can enhance relaxation.
- Relaxation positions: Sitting comfortably in a well-supported chair with your back straight and feet flat on the floor, or lying in a supine position.

Relaxation Exercise

Take a deep breath. As you exhale, close your eyes. Continue breathing slowly and fully. (Pause.) Scan your body and pinpoint tense areas. Focus on sending deep relaxation to each individual area. (Pause.) With each inhalation, relax further. As you exhale, the tension releases and exits your body, enabling you to feel peaceful and serene. Let go of any extraneous thoughts and give yourself permission to experience inner peace and stillness. (Pause.) Focus on your breathing. Begin to count down slowly from 20 to 1, taking a full breath with each number. Allow yourself to enter a deeper level of tranquility.

This section contains the formulas and exercises to use the mind for life empowerment.

THE ESSENCE OF HEALING

If a person is looking for a long-lasting solution to a problem, it requires the total incorporation of the body/mind/spirit connection. If an individual merely works on the physical level, the result of the healing effect may only be temporary. For example, receiving a massage is a wonderful way to improve the feeling of well-being. Stress and tension are removed, muscles feel looser and more limber, and the mind is more at ease. But the improvement may only last a few days at best unless a longer-term program is instituted that includes the person's mental, emotional, and spiritual parts, in addition to the physical. To accomplish this, an important step is to initiate a forgiveness effort with a goal to completely let go of all unresolved resentment, anger, and hurt. As we forgive others, so will we be forgiven. Another important part of healing is increasing the love for ourselves and improving our attitude. The *Forgiveness, Loving Yourself, Creating Good Karma, Higher Consciousness,* and *Attitude Is Most Important* formulas will be especially helpful. The body wants to be healthy and it is up to us to provide what it needs to heal itself.

FORMULAS

APPRECIATION

It is important to appreciate everything we have in life. It is unfortunate that too many people wait for a tragedy to occur or to be on their deathbeds before experiencing feelings of contrition and regret for not having enjoyed the closeness of loved ones.

- Select one of these methods: application, inhaler, or mist spray; and use a formula.

- Do the relaxation exercise on page 27. Allow yourself to reach a peaceful, quiet state. On a sheet of paper, make a list of the people you need to spend more time with and appreciate more. Next to each name, list what you'd like to express in words and also in action to the person and the amount of time you plan to spend with them. After being with the person, write down the results of how this exercise was beneficial.

- Repeat this exercise often. Each session should be about 20 to 30 minutes.

Appreciation—Application

Apply one of these formulas to the wrists, upper chest, and back of the neck, until the oil has been fully absorbed into the skin. Bring your wrists close to your nose and breathe the vapors in deeply. When done, if you wish, dab on cornstarch to dry off any remaining oil.

Rosewood	3 drops
Allspice Berry	3 drops
Lemon	3 drops
Ylang-Ylang	1 drop
Carrier Oil	2 teaspoons (10 ml)

Allspice Berry	3 drops
Petitgrain	2 drops
Neroli	2 drops
Lemongrass	2 drops
Patchouli	1 drop
Carrier Oil	2 teaspoons (10 ml)

Litsea Cubeba	3 drops
Rosewood	3 drops
Geranium	2 drops
Vanilla (CO_2)	2 drops
Carrier Oil	2 teaspoons (10 ml)

Sandalwood	3 drops
Lemongrass	2 drops
Tangerine	2 drops
Cumin	2 drops
Vanilla (CO_2)	1 drop
Carrier Oil	2 teaspoons (10 ml)

Lemon	3 drops
Petitgrain	3 drops
Amyris	2 drops
Clove Bud	1 drop
Neroli	1 drop
Carrier Oil	2 teaspoons (10 ml)

Petitgrain	3 drops
Neroli	3 drops
Lemongrass	2 drops
Cedarwood (Atlas)	1 drop
Orange	1 drop
Carrier Oil	2 teaspoons (10 ml)

Tangerine	3 drops
Orange	2 drops
Grapefruit	2 drops
Neroli	2 drops
Cedarwood (Atlas)	1 drop
Carrier Oil	2 teaspoons (10 ml)

Bergamot	3 drops
Citronella	3 drops
Sandalwood	2 drops
Vanilla (CO_2)	2 drops
Carrier Oil	2 teaspoons (10 ml)

Appreciation—Inhaler

Choose one of these formulas. Combine the essential oils in a small glass bottle with a wide opening. Inhale the vapors slowly and deeply. Then tightly cap the bottle after using.

Tangerine	10 drops
Lemongrass	10 drops
Patchouli	5 drops

Orange	10 drops
Grapefruit	10 drops
Clove Bud	5 drops
Ylang-Ylang	5 drops
Cedarwood (Atlas)	5 drops

Bergamot	10 drops
Eucalyptus Citriodora	10 drops
Geranium	10 drops
Vanilla (CO_2)	5 drops

Grapefruit	10 drops
Citronella	10 drops
Tangerine	10 drops
Ginger	5 drops
Cedarwood (Atlas)	5 drops

Tangerine	13 drops
Bergamot	12 drops
Litsea Cubeba	10 drops
Patchouli	5 drops

Rosewood	10 drops
Lemon	10 drops
Lemongrass	10 drops
Vanilla (CO_2)	5 drops

Appreciation—Mist Spray

Choose one of these formulas. Fill a fine-mist spray bottle with 2 ounces (60 ml) of purified water, add the essential oils, tighten the cap, and shake well. Mist numerous times over the head with eyes closed. Breathe the vapors in slowly and deeply.

Petitgrain	18 drops
Rosewood	15 drops
Tangerine	15 drops
Lemon	15 drops
Grapefruit	12 drops
Pure Water	2 ounces (60 ml)

Litsea Cubeba	22 drops
Bergamot	18 drops
Ylang-Ylang	15 drops
Petitgrain	10 drops
Cedarwood (Atlas)	10 drops
Pure Water	2 ounces (60 ml)

Tangerine	18 drops
Lemon	15 drops
Eucalyptus Citriodora	12 drops
Orange	10 drops
Peppermint	10 drops
Patchouli	5 drops
Geranium	5 drops
Pure Water	2 ounces (60 ml)

Lime	15 drops
Grapefruit	15 drops
Rosewood	15 drops
Allspice Berry	12 drops
Tangerine	8 drops
Citronella	5 drops
Guaiacwood	5 drops
Pure Water	2 ounces (60 ml)

ATTITUDE IS MOST IMPORTANT

The majority of people will agree that if we improve our attitude, we will improve our life. If this is so obvious, then why don't more people have a better attitude? We have the power to choose the attitude we want to have. We decide how we see fit to interact with others, and how courteous, honorable, trustworthy, responsible, helpful, considerate, kind, cooperative, and caring we want to be. A good attitude is of great benefit to all of us.

- Select one of these methods: application, inhaler, or mist spray; and use a formula.

- Do the relaxation exercise on page 27. Allow yourself to reach a peaceful, quiet state and reflect on how you can improve your attitude. Write your thoughts down on a sheet of paper and start putting them into action.

- Repeat this exercise regularly. Each session should be about 20 to 30 minutes.

Attitude Is Most Important—Application

Apply one of these formulas to the wrists, upper chest, and back of the neck, until the oil has been fully absorbed into the skin. Bring your wrists close to your nose and breathe the vapors in deeply. When done, if you wish, dab on cornstarch to dry off any remaining oil.

Helichrysum	4 drops
Lemon	4 drops
Neroli	2 drops
Carrier Oil	2 teaspoons (10 ml)

Mandarin	5 drops
Helichrysum	3 drops
Vanilla (CO_2)	2 drops
Carrier Oil	2 teaspoons (10 ml)

Frankincense	3 drops
Neroli	3 drops
Mandarin	3 drops
Sandalwood	1 drop
Carrier Oil	2 teaspoons (10 ml)

Helichrysum	4 drops
Spearmint	3 drops
Champaca Flower	3 drops
Carrier Oil	2 teaspoons (10 ml)

Champaca Flower	4 drops
Vanilla (CO_2)	3 drops
Ginger	2 drops
Sandalwood	1 drop
Carrier Oil	2 teaspoons (10 ml)

Spruce	4 drops
Vanilla (CO_2)	3 drops
Sandalwood	3 drops
Carrier Oil	2 teaspoons (10 ml)

Tangerine	4 drops
Spearmint	3 drops
Vanilla (CO_2)	2 drops
Ginger	1 drop
Carrier Oil	2 teaspoons (10 ml)

Spruce	4 drops
Helichrysum	3 drops
Tangerine	3 drops
Carrier Oil	2 teaspoons (10 ml)

Tangerine	4 drops
Lemon Myrtle	2 drops
Vanilla (CO_2)	2 drops
Amyris	2 drops
Carrier Oil	2 teaspoons (10 ml)

Neroli	3 drops
Lemon Myrtle	2 drops
Champaca Flower	2 drops
Vetiver	2 drops
Frankincense	1 drop
Carrier Oil	2 teaspoons (10 ml)

Attitude Is Most Important—Inhaler

Choose one of these formulas. Combine the essential oils in a small glass bottle with a wide opening. Inhale the vapors slowly and deeply. Then tightly cap the bottle after using.

Lemon	10 drops
Orange	10 drops
Spearmint	10 drops

Litsea Cubeba	10 drops
Orange	10 drops
Lemon	10 drops
Patchouli	5 drops

Tangerine	15 drops
Neroli	10 drops
Patchouli	5 drops

Grapefruit	20 drops
Orange	15 drops
Clove Bud	5 drops
Amyris	5 drops

Attitude Is Most Important—Mist Spray

Choose one of these formulas. Fill a fine-mist spray bottle with 2 ounces (60 ml) of purified water, add the essential oils, tighten the cap, and shake well. Mist numerous times over the head with eyes closed. Breathe the vapors in slowly and deeply.

Orange	25 drops
Petitgrain	20 drops
Lemon	20 drops
Helichrysum	10 drops
Pure Water	2 ounces (60 ml)

Litsea Cubeba	25 drops
Grapefruit	20 drops
Clove Bud	20 drops
Patchouli	10 drops
Pure Water	2 ounces (60 ml)

Tangerine	20 drops
Grapefruit	20 drops
Spearmint	15 drops
Lemon	15 drops
Patchouli	5 drops
Pure Water	2 ounces (60 ml)

Litsea Cubeba	25 drops
Orange	25 drops
Spruce	15 drops
Ginger	10 drops
Pure Water	2 ounces (60 ml)

CREATING GOOD KARMA

- Select one of these methods: application, inhaler, or mist spray; and use a formula.

- Do the relaxation exercise on page 27. Allow yourself to reach a peaceful, quiet state and think about the wrongdoings you've done in the past to yourself and others. Write them down on a sheet of paper and reflect on what actions you can take to correct each one of them and make a note of it. Then see what additional insight you can come up with to do to improve your karma. After the session, be sure to carry out your plan of action.

- Repeat this exercise and continue to receive insight. Each session should be about 20 to 30 minutes.

Creating Good Karma—Application

Apply one of these formulas to the wrists, upper chest, and back of the neck, until the oil has been fully absorbed into the skin. Bring your wrists close to your nose and breathe the vapors in deeply. When done, if you wish, dab on cornstarch to dry off any remaining oil.

Frankincense	3 drops
Fir Needles	3 drops
Vanilla (CO_2)	2 drops
Cedarwood (Atlas)	2 drops
Carrier Oil	2 teaspoons (10 ml)

Rosewood	3 drops
Myrtle	3 drops
Amyris	2 drops
Spearmint	2 drops
Carrier Oil	2 teaspoons (10 ml)

Spruce	4 drops
Guaiacwood	4 drops
Lemon	2 drops
Carrier Oil	2 teaspoons (10 ml)

Spruce	3 drops
Lemon	3 drops
Tangerine	2 drops
Cedarwood (Atlas)	2 drops
Carrier Oil	2 teaspoons (10 ml)

Fir Needles	3 drops
Juniper Berry	3 drops
Frankincense	2 drops
Litsea Cubeba	2 drops
Carrier Oil	2 teaspoons (10 ml)

Litsea Cubeba	4 drops
Guaiacwood	4 drops
Ginger	2 drops
Carrier Oil	2 teaspoons (10 ml)

Fir Needles	3 drops
Mandarin	3 drops
Myrtle	2 drops
Spearmint	2 drops
Carrier Oil	2 teaspoons (10 ml)

Lemon	3 drops
Guaiacwood	3 drops
Neroli	3 drops
Ginger	1 drop
Carrier Oil	2 teaspoons (10 ml)

Frankincense	4 drops
Helichrysum	2 drops
Spruce	2 drops
Lemon Myrtle	2 drops
Carrier Oil	2 teaspoons (10 ml)

Spruce	3 drops
Amyris	3 drops
Anise	2 drops
Lemon Myrtle	2 drops
Carrier Oil	2 teaspoons (10 ml)

Creating Good Karma—Inhaler

Choose one of these formulas. Combine the essential oils in a small glass bottle with a wide opening. Inhale the vapors slowly and deeply. Then tightly cap the bottle after using.

Frankincense	10 drops
Fir Needles	10 drops
Cedarwood (Atlas)	10 drops
Vanilla (CO_2)	5 drops

Rosewood	10 drops
Myrtle	10 drops
Spearmint	7 drops
Amyris	5 drops

Spruce	15 drops
Guaiacwood	15 drops
Lemon	10 drops

Spruce	15 drops
Lemon	10 drops
Tangerine	10 drops
Cedarwood (Atlas)	5 drops

Fir Needles	13 drops
Frankincense	12 drops
Litsea Cubeba	10 drops

Litsea Cubeba	15 drops
Guaiacwood	10 drops
Ginger	5 drops

Creating Good Karma—Mist Spray

Choose one of these formulas. Fill a fine-mist spray bottle with 2 ounces (60 ml) of purified water, add the essential oils, tighten the cap, and shake well. Mist numerous times over the head with eyes closed. Breathe the vapors in slowly and deeply.

Frankincense	20 drops
Ravensara Aromatica	18 drops
Juniper Berry	17 drops
Eucalyptus Citriodora	15 drops
Amyris	5 drops
Pure Water	2 ounces (60 ml)

Fir Needles	18 drops
Rosewood	18 drops
Clove Bud	10 drops
Myrtle	10 drops
Litsea Cubeba	10 drops
Guaiacwood	9 drops
Pure Water	2 ounces (60 ml)

Spruce	20 drops
Fir Needles	18 drops
Orange	17 drops
Cedarwood (Atlas)	15 drops
Lemon	5 drops
Pure Water	2 ounces (60 ml)

Spruce	18 drops
Pine	15 drops
Orange	15 drops
Litsea Cubeba	15 drops
Cedarwood (Atlas)	12 drops
Pure Water	2 ounces (60 ml)

DO UNTO OTHERS

Do unto others as you would have them do unto you. Be the person you would like to see others be toward you.

- ❧ By doing good unto others we improve our own outlook.

- ❧ If you want to be forgiven—be forgiving.

- ❧ If you want to be loved—be loving.

- ❧ If you want to be understood—be understanding.

- ❧ If you want peace—be a peacemaker.

- ❧ If you want kindness—be kind.

- ❧ If you want justice—don't be indifferent when injustice is done to others.

- ❧ If you want cooperation—be cooperative.

- ❧ If you want respect—be respectful.

- ❧ If you want to be appreciated—express appreciation to others.

- Select one of these methods: application, inhaler, or mist spray; and use a formula.

- Do the relaxation exercise on page 27. Allow yourself to reach a peaceful, quiet state. Then reflect on if you are treating other people as you would like to be treated yourself. On a sheet of paper, write down the improvements you need to make when interacting with other people.

- Repeat this exercise as often as necessary. Each session should be about 20 to 30 minutes.

Do Unto Others—Application

Apply one of these formulas to the wrists, upper chest, and back of the neck, until the oil has been fully absorbed into the skin. Bring your wrists close to your nose and breathe the vapors in deeply. When done, if you wish, dab on cornstarch to dry off any remaining oil.

Spruce	3 drops
Lemon	3 drops
Mandarin	2 drops
Vanilla (CO_2)	2 drops
Carrier Oil	2 teaspoons (10 ml)
Spruce	4 drops
Clary Sage	3 drops
Vanilla (CO_2)	3 drops
Carrier Oil	2 teaspoons (10 ml)
Clary Sage	3 drops
Lavender	3 drops
Mandarin	2 drops
Cedarwood (Atlas)	2 drops
Carrier Oil	2 teaspoons (10 ml)
Helichrysum	3 drops
Clary Sage	3 drops
Neroli	2 drops
Cedarwood (Atlas)	2 drops
Carrier Oil	2 teaspoons (10 ml)
Helichrysum	4 drops
Mandarin	2 drops
Rosewood	2 drops
Vetiver	2 drops
Carrier Oil	2 teaspoons (10 ml)
Helichrysum	3 drops
Champaca Flower	3 drops
Rosewood	2 drops
Vanilla (CO_2)	2 drops
Carrier Oil	2 teaspoons (10 ml)
Champaca Flower	4 drops
Neroli	2 drops
Rosewood	2 drops
Sandalwood	2 drops
Carrier Oil	2 teaspoons (10 ml)

Clary Sage	3 drops
Sandalwood	3 drops
Clove Bud	2 drops
Rose	2 drops
Carrier Oil	2 teaspoons (10 ml)

Do Unto Others—Inhaler

Choose one of these formulas. Combine the essential oils in a small glass bottle with a wide opening. Inhale the vapors slowly and deeply. Then tightly cap the bottle after using.

Spruce	20 drops
Mandarin	10 drops
Vanilla (CO_2)	10 drops

Mandarin	20 drops
Neroli	10 drops
Vetiver	5 drops

Clary Sage	15 drops
Champaca Flower	15 drops
Rosewood	10 drops

Helichrysum	10 drops
Spruce	10 drops
Lemon	10 drops
Cedarwood (Atlas)	3 drops

Do Unto Others—Mist Spray

Choose one of these formulas. Fill a fine-mist spray bottle with 2 ounces (60 ml) of purified water, add the essentials oils, tighten the cap, and shake well. Mist numerous times over the head with eyes closed. Breathe the vapors in slowly and deeply.

Spruce	25 drops
Lemon	25 drops
Cedarwood (Atlas)	15 drops
Rosewood	10 drops
Pure Water	2 ounces (60 ml)

Spruce	28 drops
Clary Sage	22 drops
Rosewood	15 drops
Clove Bud	10 drops
Pure Water	2 ounces (60 ml)

Lavender	25 drops
Clary Sage	25 drops
Mandarin	20 drops
Vetiver	5 drops
Pure Water	2 ounces (60 ml)

Mandarin	25 drops
Rosewood	23 drops
Lemon	22 drops
Vanilla (CO_2)	5 drops
Pure Water	2 ounces (60 ml)

EVERY EXPERIENCE IS A TEACHER

Instead of acquiring guilt or blaming someone else for things that go wrong, let every experience be a learning lesson, so that the bad experiences are not repeated. We don't have to go through life experiencing the same lessons over and over again, if we learn from it the first time.

- Select one of these methods: application, inhaler, or mist spray; and use a formula.

- Do the relaxation exercise on page 27. Allow yourself to reach a peaceful, quiet state. Then focus on the different experiences you are having and what you can learn from each one. Write down on a sheet of paper what you've come up with and how this can help you from now on.

- Repeat this exercise whenever necessary. Each session should be about 20 to 30 minutes.

Every Experience Is a Teacher— Application

Apply one of these formulas to the wrists, upper chest, and back of the neck, until the oil has been fully absorbed into the skin. Bring your wrists close to your nose and breathe the vapors in deeply. When done, if you wish, dab on cornstarch to dry off any remaining oil.

Tangerine	3 drops
Neroli	3 drops
Galbanum	2 drops
Lemon Myrtle	2 drops
Carrier Oil	2 teaspoons (10 ml)

Helichrysum	3 drops
Dill	3 drops
Vanilla (CO_2)	2 drops
Anise	2 drops
Carrier Oil	2 teaspoons (10 ml)

Helichrysum	3 drops
Spruce	3 drops
Fir Needles	2 drops
Orange	2 drops
Carrier Oil	2 teaspoons (10 ml)

Spruce	3 drops
Neroli	3 drops
Myrtle	2 drops
Rosewood	2 drops
Carrier Oil	2 teaspoons (10 ml)

Chamomile (Roman)	3 drops
Vanilla (CO_2)	3 drops
Galbanum	3 drops
Nutmeg	1 drop
Carrier Oil	2 teaspoons (10 ml)

Tangerine	3 drops
Galbanum	3 drops
Cedarwood (Atlas)	3 drops
Nutmeg	1 drop
Carrier Oil	2 teaspoons (10 ml)

Dill	3 drops
Spruce	3 drops
Neroli	2 drops
Chamomile (Roman)	2 drops
Carrier Oil	2 teaspoons (10 ml)

Chamomile (Roman)	4 drops
Champaca Flower	4 drops
Galbanum	2 drops
Carrier Oil	2 teaspoons (10 ml)

Every Experience Is a Teacher—Inhaler

Choose one of these formulas. Combine the essential oils in a small glass bottle with a wide opening. Inhale the vapors slowly and deeply. Then tightly cap the bottle after using.

Tangerine	25 drops
Cedarwood (Atlas)	10 drops

Neroli	15 drops
Dill	5 drops

Chamomile (Roman)	15 drops
Citronella	5 drops

Spruce	20 drops
Anise	5 drops

Every Experience Is a Teacher—Mist Spray

Choose one of these formulas. Fill a fine-mist spray bottle with 2 ounces (60 ml) of purified water, add the essentials oils, tighten the cap, and shake well. Mist numerous times over the head with eyes closed. Breathe the vapors in slowly and deeply.

Spruce	20 drops
Dill	15 drops
Tangerine	15 drops
Myrtle	15 drops
Cedarwood (Atlas)	10 drops
Pure Water	2 ounces (60 ml)

Chamomile (Roman)	20 drops
Citronella	20 drops
Fir Needles	20 drops
Rosewood	15 drops
Pure Water	2 ounces (60 ml)

Tangerine	20 drops
Myrtle	15 drops
Dill	15 drops
Citronella	15 drops
Cedarwood (Atlas)	10 drops
Pure Water	2 ounces (60 ml)

Spruce	25 drops
Citronella	20 drops
Galbanum	15 drops
Nutmeg	5 drops
Vanilla (CO_2)	5 drops
Myrtle	5 drops
Pure Water	2 ounces (60 ml)

Orange	25 drops
Chamomile (Roman)	20 drops
Dill	15 drops
Galbanum	15 drops
Pure Water	2 ounces (60 ml)

Tangerine	25 drops
Fir Needles	25 drops
Spruce	15 drops
Vanilla (CO_2)	10 drops
Pure Water	2 ounces (60 ml)

FORGIVENESS

- Select one of these methods: application, inhaler, or mist spray; and use a formula.

- Do the relaxation exercise on page 27. Allow yourself to reach a peaceful, quiet state. Then focus on letting go of the hurt and resentment you are carrying around. On a sheet of paper, make a list of all the people you need to forgive and keep doing the exercise as often as you can until you free yourself. Only you have the power to accomplish this great feat. Remember, forgiveness helps the forgiver.

- Each session should be about 20 to 30 minutes.

Forgiveness—Application

Apply one of these formulas to the wrists, upper chest, and back of the neck, until the oil has been fully absorbed into the skin. Bring your wrists close to your nose and breathe the vapors in deeply. When done, if you wish, dab on corn-starch to dry off any remaining oil.

Spruce	4 drops
Cinnamon Leaf	3 drops
Tangerine	3 drops
Carrier Oil	2 teaspoons (10 ml)

Fir Needles	4 drops
Cinnamon Leaf	3 drops
Frankincense	3 drops
Carrier Oil	2 teaspoons (10 ml)

Lemon	3 drops
Fir Needles	3 drops
Spruce	3 drops
Cedarwood (Atlas)	1 drop
Carrier Oil	2 teaspoons (10 ml)

Lemon	3 drops
Spruce	3 drops
Helichrysum	2 drops
Cinnamon Leaf	2 drops
Carrier Oil	2 teaspoons (10 ml)

Neroli	3 drops
Rosewood	3 drops
Spruce	2 drops
Cardamom	2 drops
Carrier Oil	2 teaspoons (10 ml)

Mandarin	3 drops
Spruce	3 drops
Cedarwood (Atlas)	3 drops
Helichrysum	1 drop
Carrier Oil	2 teaspoons (10 ml)

Lemon	2 drops
Cinnamon Leaf	2 drops
Vanilla (CO_2)	2 drops
Helichrysum	2 drops
Neroli	2 drops
Carrier Oil	2 teaspoons (10 ml)

Vanilla (CO_2)	4 drops
Neroli	3 drops
Tangerine	2 drops
Cumin	1 drop
Carrier Oil	2 teaspoons (10 ml)

Spruce	4 drops
Rosewood	3 drops
Vanilla (CO_2)	3 drops
Carrier Oil	2 teaspoons (10 ml)

Rosewood	3 drops
Champaca Flower	3 drops
Tangerine	2 drops
Helichrysum	2 drops
Carrier Oil	2 teaspoons (10 ml)

Forgiveness—Inhaler

Choose one of these formulas. Combine the essential oils in a small glass bottle with a wide opening. Inhale the vapors slowly and deeply. Then tightly cap the bottle after using.

Spruce	20 drops
Orange	15 drops

Spruce	15 drops
Spearmint	15 drops
Vanilla (CO_2)	8 drops
Orange	7 drops

Spruce	20 drops
Cardamom	10 drops

Lemon	15 drops
Tangerine	15 drops
Fir Needles	5 drops
Cedarwood (Atlas)	5 drops

Forgiveness—Mist Spray

Choose one of these formulas. Fill a fine-mist spray bottle with 2 ounces (60 ml) of purified water, add the essentials oils, tighten the cap, and shake well. Mist numerous times over the head with eyes closed. Breathe the vapors in slowly and deeply.

Spruce	20 drops
Allspice Berry	20 drops
Tangerine	13 drops
Spearmint	12 drops
Cinnamon Leaf	10 drops
Pure Water	2 ounces (60 ml)

Chamomile (Roman)	25 drops
Frankincense	20 drops
Lemon	20 drops
Orange	10 drops
Pure Water	2 ounces (60 ml)

Lemon	30 drops
Spruce	30 drops
Frankincense	15 drops
Pure Water	2 ounces (60 ml)

Fir Needles	40 drops
Helichrysum	20 drops
Tangerine	15 drops
Pure Water	2 ounces (60 ml)

Spruce	40 drops
Tangerine	20 drops
Fir Needles	10 drops
Cedarwood (Atlas)	5 drops
Pure Water	2 ounces (60 ml)

Tangerine	25 drops
Lemon	25 drops
Cardamom	13 drops
Chamomile (Roman)	12 drops
Pure Water	2 ounces (60 ml)

Spruce	40 drops
Lemon Myrtle	25 drops
Cedarwood (Atlas)	10 drops
Pure Water	2 ounces (60 ml)

Lemon Myrtle	20 drops
Fir Needles	20 drops
Clove Bud	18 drops
Tangerine	12 drops
Patchouli	5 drops
Pure Water	2 ounces (60 ml)

HIGHER CONSCIOUSNESS

Please see pages 20–21; make a list of the virtues you need to improve on, and do the following exercise.

- Select one of these methods: application, inhaler, or mist spray; and use a formula.

- Do the relaxation exercise on page 27. Allow yourself to reach a peaceful, quiet state. Write down on a sheet of paper, how you plan to improve and practice each virtue you have listed. Then every week assess the progress you have made and write down your results.

- Repeat this exercise as often as necessary. Each session should be about 20 to 30 minutes.

Higher Consciousness—Application

Apply one of these formulas to the wrists, upper chest, and back of the neck, until the oil has been fully absorbed into the skin. Bring your wrists close to your nose and breathe the vapors in deeply. When done, if you wish, dab on cornstarch to dry off any remaining oil.

Frankincense	3 drops
Spruce	3 drops
Spikenard	3 drops
Cinnamon Leaf	1 drop
Carrier Oil	2 teaspoons (10 ml)

Fir Needles	3 drops
Spruce	3 drops
Basil (Sweet)	2 drops
Vanilla (CO_2)	2 drops
Carrier Oil	2 teaspoons (10 ml)

Lemon	3 drops
Grapefruit	3 drops
Frankincense	2 drops
Cinnamon Leaf	2 drops
Carrier Oil	2 teaspoons (10 ml)

Frankincense	3 drops
Basil (Sweet)	3 drops
Cedarwood (Atlas)	2 drops
Cinnamon Leaf	2 drops
Carrier Oil	2 teaspoons (10 ml)

Myrtle	3 drops
Spruce	3 drops
Guaiacwood	2 drops
Mandarin	2 drops
Carrier Oil	2 teaspoons (10 ml)

Lemon	3 drops
Spruce	3 drops
Cedarwood (Atlas)	2 drops
Basil (Sweet)	2 drops
Carrier Oil	2 teaspoons (10 ml)

Helichrysum	4 drops
Guaiacwood	2 drops
Lemon	2 drops
Citronella	2 drops
Carrier Oil	2 teaspoons (10 ml)

Helichrysum	4 drops
Sage (Spanish)	2 drops
Cabreuva	2 drops
Vanilla (CO_2)	2 drops
Carrier Oil	2 teaspoons (10 ml)

Spruce	3 drops
Helichrysum	3 drops
Lemon	3 drops
Cedarwood (Atlas)	1 drop
Carrier Oil	2 teaspoons (10 ml)

Helichrysum	4 drops
Spruce	4 drops
Vanilla (CO_2)	2 drops
Carrier Oil	2 teaspoons (10 ml)

Higher Consciousness—Inhaler

Choose one of these formulas. Combine the essential oils in a small glass bottle with a wide opening. Inhale the vapors slowly and deeply. Then tightly cap the bottle after using.

Helichrysum	20 drops
Sage (Spanish)	10 drops
Cabreuva	10 drops
Vanilla (CO_2)	5 drops

Helichrysum	10 drops
Spruce	10 drops
Lemon	10 drops

Fir Needles	15 drops
Frankincense	10 drops
Cinnamon Leaf	5 drops
Spearmint	5 drops

Spruce	20 drops
Basil (Sweet)	5 drops
Guaiacwood	5 drops
Vanilla (CO_2)	5 drops

Lemon	10 drops
Spruce	10 drops
Helichrysum	10 drops
Cedarwood (Atlas)	5 drops

Fir Needles	13 drops
Lemon	13 drops
Frankincense	12 drops

Higher Consciousness—Mist Spray

Choose one of these formulas. Fill a fine-mist spray bottle with 2 ounces (60 ml) of purified water, add the essential oils, tighten the cap, and shake well. Mist numerous times over the head with eyes closed. Breathe the vapors in slowly and deeply.

Litsea Cubeba	15 drops
Frankincense	15 drops
Spruce	15 drops
Basil (Sweet)	10 drops
Amyris	10 drops
Vetiver	10 drops
Pure Water	2 ounces (60 ml)

Juniper Berry	16 drops
Cedarwood (Atlas)	15 drops
Helichrysum	15 drops
Cypress	14 drops
Citronella	10 drops
Spearmint	5 drops
Pure Water	2 ounces (60 ml)

Lemon	20 drops
Myrtle	15 drops
Basil (Sweet)	15 drops
Spearmint	15 drops
Sage (Spanish)	10 drops
Pure Water	2 ounces (60 ml)

Fir Needles	20 drops
Helichrysum	20 drops
Litsea Cubeba	15 drops
Cedarwood (Atlas)	10 drops
Spearmint	10 drops
Pure Water	2 ounces (60 ml)

IMPROVEMENT

Each day we should be making progress to become a better person. Life continually gives us experiences to help us grow in our development. It is important we take advantage and learn from every opportunity we get.

- Select one of these methods: application, inhaler, or mist spray; and use a formula.

- Do the relaxation exercise on page 27. Allow yourself to reach a peaceful, quiet state. Write down on a sheet of paper, the constructive criticism people have given you and the improvements you intend to make. Then reflect on the specific changes you are considering. Afterward, write a plan of action for each change. Each week assess your progress and the benefits you have derived from the improvements.

- Repeat this exercise whenever necessary. Each session should be about 20 to 30 minutes.

Improvement—Application

Apply one of these formulas to the wrists, upper chest, and back of the neck, until the oil has been fully absorbed into the skin. Bring your wrists close to your nose and breathe the vapors in deeply. When done, if you wish, dab on cornstarch to dry off any remaining oil.

Rosewood	4 drops
Tangerine	2 drops
Lemon	2 drops
Cardamom	2 drops
Carrier Oil	2 teaspoons (10 ml)

Litsea Cubeba	3 drops
Geranium	2 drops
Cedarwood (Atlas)	2 drops
Cardamom	2 drops
Spearmint	1 drop
Carrier Oil	2 teaspoons (10 ml)

Frankincense	3 drops
Vanilla (CO_2)	2 drops
Cardamom	2 drops
Cedarwood (Atlas)	2 drops
Spearmint	1 drop
Carrier Oil	2 teaspoons (10 ml)

Rosewood	2 drops
Vanilla (CO_2)	2 drops
Orange	2 drops
Helichrysum	2 drops
Cinnamon Leaf	2 drops
Carrier Oil	2 teaspoons (10 ml)

Helichrysum	4 drops
Orange	4 drops
Cinnamon Leaf	2 drops
Carrier Oil	2 teaspoons (10 ml)

Orange	3 drops
Chamomile (Roman)	3 drops
Cardamom	2 drops
Cedarwood (Atlas)	2 drops
Carrier Oil	2 teaspoons (10 ml)

Improvement—Inhaler

Choose one of these formulas. Combine the essential oils in a small glass bottle with a wide opening. Inhale the vapors slowly and deeply. Then tightly cap the bottle after using.

Tangerine	15 drops
Litsea Cubeba	15 drops
Cardamom	10 drops

Spruce	13 drops
Frankincense	12 drops
Cardamom	10 drops

Litsea Cubeba	10 drops
Frankincense	10 drops
Spearmint	10 drops

Helichrysum	13 drops
Spruce	10 drops
Lemon	10 drops

Improvement—Mist Spray

Choose one of these formulas. Fill a fine-mist spray bottle with 2 ounces (60 ml) of purified water, add the essential oils, tighten the cap, and shake well. Mist numerous times over the head with eyes closed. Breathe the vapors in slowly and deeply.

Orange	17 drops
Cardamom	17 drops
Tangerine	16 drops
Myrtle	15 drops
Cedarwood (Atlas)	10 drops
Pure Water	2 ounces (60 ml)

Tangerine	20 drops
Helichrysum	18 drops
Cardamom	17 drops
Guaiacwood	10 drops
Chamomile (Roman)	10 drops
Pure Water	2 ounces (60 ml)

Cedarwood (Atlas)	17 drops
Myrtle	17 drops
Cardamom	17 drops
Lavender	15 drops
Litsea Cubeba	9 drops
Pure Water	2 ounces (60 ml)

Lemon	14 drops
Grapefruit	14 drops
Tangerine	14 drops
Spruce	14 drops
Guaiacwood	12 drops
Orange	7 drops
Pure Water	2 ounces (60 ml)

INTROSPECTION

- Select one of these methods: application, inhaler, or mist spray; and use a formula.

- Do the relaxation exercise on page 27. Allow yourself to reach a peaceful, quiet state; then take a closer look at yourself. On a personal level, compare how your daily actions measure up to your moral values and the principles you stand for. On an interpersonal level, examine how you honor your promises, commitments, and responsibilities to the people in your life. Write down on a sheet of paper, your insights on a personal level and the planned changes and actions to be taken. Then, on another sheet of paper, do the same for the insights received on an interpersonal level, and the changes and actions you plan to take.

- Repeat this exercise as many times as you feel necessary. Each session should be about 20 to 30 minutes.

Introspection—Application

Apply one of these formulas to the wrists, upper chest, and back of the neck, until the oil has been fully absorbed into the skin. Bring your wrists close to your nose and breathe the vapors in deeply. When done, if you wish, dab on cornstarch to dry off any remaining oil.

Lemon	3 drops
Frankincense	3 drops
Spruce	2 drops
Tangerine	2 drops
Carrier Oil	2 teaspoons (10 ml)

Orange	3 drops
Spikenard	3 drops
Cajeput	2 drops
Spruce	2 drops
Carrier Oil	2 teaspoons (10 ml)

Tangerine	4 drops
Lemon	3 drops
Frankincense	3 drops
Carrier Oil	2 teaspoons (10 ml)

Cypress	3 drops
Lemongrass	3 drops
Rosewood	2 drops
Spikenard	2 drops
Carrier Oil	2 teaspoons (10 ml)

Spruce	4 drops
Vetiver	2 drops
Lemongrass	2 drops
Cajeput	2 drops
Carrier Oil	2 teaspoons (10 ml)

Spruce	4 drops
Rosewood	3 drops
Orange	3 drops
Carrier Oil	2 teaspoons (10 ml)

Introspection—Inhaler

Choose one of these formulas. Combine the essential oils in a small glass bottle with a wide opening. Inhale the vapors slowly and deeply. Then tightly cap the bottle after using.

Spruce	12 drops
Spearmint	10 drops
Cedarwood (Atlas)	10 drops

Spruce	13 drops
Cajeput	10 drops
Neroli	7 drops

Frankincense	10 drops
Spruce	10 drops
Pine	8 drops
Vanilla (CO_2)	7 drops

Frankincense	13 drops
Litsea Cubeba	10 drops
Neroli	8 drops
Rosewood	4 drops

Frankincense	12 drops
Spruce	8 drops
Spearmint	8 drops
Lemon	5 drops

Cajeput	10 drops
Lemon	10 drops
Spruce	10 drops
Orange	10 drops

Introspection—Mist Spray

Choose one of these formulas. Fill a fine-mist spray bottle with 2 ounces (60 ml) of purified water, add the essential oils, tighten the cap, and shake well. Mist numerous times over the head with eyes closed. Breathe the vapors in slowly and deeply.

Frankincense	25 drops
Lemongrass	25 drops
Tangerine	15 drops
Vetiver	10 drops
Pure Water	2 ounces (60 ml)

Cajeput	30 drops
Lemon	30 drops
Basil (Sweet)	15 drops
Pure Water	2 ounces (60 ml)

Spruce	30 drops
Orange	25 drops
Cajeput	10 drops
Cedarwood (Atlas)	10 drops
Pure Water	2 ounces (60 ml)

Orange	20 drops
Lemon	20 drops
Frankincense	20 drops
Spruce	15 drops
Pure Water	2 ounces (60 ml)

INTUITION

An abundance of solutions exist in the universe, but they can only be found by those who seek them. If you have a decision to make and need guidance by looking within, these intuition formulas can help relax your mind and assist you in getting input.

- Select one of these methods: application, inhaler, or mist spray; and use a formula.

- Do the relaxation exercise on page 27. Allow yourself to reach a peaceful, quiet state. On a sheet of paper, list the decisions you need inner guidance on. Clear your mind of all extraneous thoughts, and write down the insights that come to you. Go over each one individually, and then later, ponder the input with one of the *Mental Concentration* formulas on pages 52–54. Write a plan of action you feel good about.

- Repeat this exercise once daily, if possible, for about 20 to 30 minutes. It may take several days or longer to get the insight you are looking for.

Intuition—Application

Apply one of these formulas to the wrists, upper chest, and back of the neck, until the oil has been fully absorbed into the skin. Bring your wrists close to your nose and breathe the vapors in deeply. When done, if you wish, dab on cornstarch to dry off any remaining oil.

Chamomile (Roman)	4 drops
Basil (Sweet)	3 drops
Mandarin	3 drops
Carrier Oil	2 teaspoons (10 ml)

Copaiba	3 drops
Neroli	3 drops
Tangerine	3 drops
Nutmeg	1 drop
Carrier Oil	2 teaspoons (10 ml)

Rosemary	2 drops
Basil (Sweet)	2 drops
Spearmint	2 drops
Cedarwood (Atlas)	2 drops
Frankincense	2 drops
Carrier Oil	2 teaspoons (10 ml)

Sage (Spanish)	3 drops
Basil (Sweet)	3 drops
Bergamot	2 drops
Allspice Berry	2 drops
Carrier Oil	2 teaspoons (10 ml)

Sage (Spanish)	3 drops
Guaiacwood	3 drops
Basil (Sweet)	2 drops
Cinnamon Leaf	2 drops
Carrier Oil	2 teaspoons (10 ml)

Mandarin	3 drops
Chamomile (Roman)	3 drops
Neroli	2 drops
Frankincense	2 drops
Carrier Oil	2 teaspoons (10 ml)

Intuition—Inhaler

Choose one of these formulas. Combine the essential oils in a small glass bottle with a wide opening. Inhale the vapors slowly and deeply. Then tightly cap the bottle after using.

Chamomile (Roman)	10 drops
Spruce	10 drops
Basil (Sweet)	10 drops
Spearmint	10 drops

Fir Needles	10 drops
Spruce	8 drops
Chamomile (Roman)	8 drops
Litsea Cubeba	8 drops
Vanilla (CO_2)	3 drops

Litsea Cubeba	10 drops
Cedarwood (Atlas)	10 drops
Anise	4 drops
Nutmeg	3 drops
Sage (Spanish)	2 drops

Frankincense	13 drops
Basil (Sweet)	8 drops
Cinnamon Leaf	8 drops
Helichrysum	8 drops

Chamomile (Roman)	11 drops
Spruce	10 drops
Basil (Sweet)	9 drops
Vanilla (CO$_2$)	5 drops

Spruce	10 drops
Clary Sage	10 drops
Chamomile (Roman)	10 drops
Lemon	5 drops

Intuition—Mist Spray

Choose one of these formulas. Fill a fine-mist spray bottle with 2 ounces (60 ml) of purified water, add the essential oils, tighten the cap, and shake well. Mist numerous times over the head with eyes closed. Breathe the vapors in slowly and deeply.

Frankincense	25 drops
Mandarin	25 drops
Allspice Berry	10 drops
Guaiacwood	10 drops
Cinnamon Leaf	5 drops
Pure Water	2 ounces (60 ml)

Chamomile (Roman)	25 drops
Frankincense	25 drops
Neroli	15 drops
Tangerine	10 drops
Pure Water	2 ounces (60 ml)

Helichrysum	20 drops
Basil (Sweet)	15 drops
Mandarin	15 drops
Cedarwood (Atlas)	15 drops
Clary Sage	10 drops
Pure Water	2 ounces (60 ml)

Orange	20 drops
Basil (Sweet)	15 drops
Clary Sage	15 drops
Guaiacwood	15 drops
Bergamot	10 drops
Pure Water	2 ounces (60 ml)

KEEP YOUR WORD

Honor your promises and commitments. Do as you say and practice what you preach. Start by honoring your word to yourself. If you tell yourself you will do something, be very disciplined about carrying it out. Maybe you've promised yourself to start exercising more, eating better, or having more discipline in your life, but you may not have kept your promise. Now is the time to become more honest with yourself and begin correcting broken promises. It is necessary to keep your word to have self-respect, confidence, and a sense of self-worthiness.

If you want to improve keeping your word, do the following:

- Select one of these methods: application, inhaler, or mist spray; and use a formula.

- Do the relaxation exercise on page 27. Allow yourself to reach a peaceful, quiet state. Then reflect on the promises you've made to yourself and other people that you haven't kept. List the promises on a sheet of paper and work on an action plan to fulfill your obligations. Keep doing the exercise as often as you can until you accomplish keeping your word.

- Each session should be about 20 to 30 minutes.

Keep Your Word—Application

Apply one of these formulas to the wrists, upper chest, and back of the neck, until the oil has been fully absorbed into the skin. Bring your wrists close to your nose and breathe the vapors in deeply. When done, if you wish, dab on cornstarch to dry off any remaining oil.

Helichrysum	3 drops
Myrtle	3 drops
Neroli	2 drops
Lemon	2 drops
Carrier Oil	2 teaspoons (10 ml)

Spruce	4 drops
Lemon	3 drops
Helichrysum	3 drops
Carrier Oil	2 teaspoons (10 ml)

Helichrysum	4 drops
Tangerine	4 drops
Ginger	2 drops
Carrier Oil	2 teaspoons (10 ml)

Sandalwood	4 drops
Tangerine	3 drops
Helichrysum	3 drops
Carrier Oil	2 teaspoons (10 ml)

Neroli	4 drops
Tangerine	4 drops
Ginger	2 drops
Carrier Oil	2 teaspoons (10 ml)

Sandalwood	5 drops
Vanilla (CO_2)	3 drops
Ginger	2 drops
Carrier Oil	2 teaspoons (10 ml)

Fir Needles	4 drops
Helichrysum	3 drops
Vanilla (CO_2)	3 drops
Carrier Oil	2 teaspoons (10 ml)

Lemon	4 drops
Vanilla (CO_2)	4 drops
Helichrysum	2 drops
Carrier Oil	2 teaspoons (10 ml)

Keep Your Word—Inhaler

Choose one of these formulas. Combine the essential oils in a small glass bottle with a wide opening. Inhale the vapors slowly and deeply. Then tightly cap the bottle after using.

Spruce	20 drops
Tangerine	20 drops

Orange	25 drops
Myrtle	10 drops
Ginger	5 drops

Myrtle	10 drops
Chamomile (Roman)	10 drops
Tangerine	10 drops
Cedarwood (Atlas)	5 drops

Lemon	20 drops
Neroli	5 drops
Cedarwood (Atlas)	5 drops
Spruce	5 drops

Tangerine	20 drops
Helichrysum	10 drops
Ginger	5 drops

Chamomile (Roman)	15 drops
Lemon	15 drops
Ginger	5 drops

Keep Your Word—Mist Spray

Choose one of these formulas. Fill a fine-mist spray bottle with 2 ounces (60 ml) of purified water, add the essential oils, tighten the cap, and shake well. Mist numerous times over the head with eyes closed. Breathe the vapors in slowly and deeply.

Lemon	20 drops
Petitgrain	20 drops
Tangerine	20 drops
Ginger	15 drops
Pure Water	2 ounces (60 ml)

Lemon	25 drops
Myrtle	20 drops
Spruce	15 drops
Tangerine	15 drops
Pure Water	2 ounces (60 ml)

Lemon	20 drops
Grapefruit	20 drops
Rosewood	15 drops
Orange	10 drops
Cedarwood (Atlas)	10 drops
Pure Water	2 ounces (60 ml)

Chamomile (Roman)	20 drops
Orange	20 drops
Lemon	20 drops
Cedarwood (Atlas)	15 drops
Pure Water	2 ounces (60 ml)

Orange	25 drops
Lemon	25 drops
Chamomile (Roman)	15 drops
Ginger	10 drops
Pure Water	2 ounces (60 ml)

Lemon	30 drops
Grapefruit	15 drops
Helichrysum	15 drops
Ginger	15 drops
Pure Water	2 ounces (60 ml)

Grapefruit	15 drops
Petitgrain	15 drops
Helichrysum	15 drops
Orange	15 drops
Ginger	10 drops
Cedarwood (Atlas)	5 drops
Pure Water	2 ounces (60 ml)

Spruce	30 drops
Grapefruit	20 drops
Tangerine	15 drops
Cedarwood (Atlas)	10 drops
Pure Water	2 ounces (60 ml)

LOVING YOURSELF

Think of a person you have had great love for. Think of how wonderful and joyous you felt being around this person. Now, how about feeling the same love for yourself? You're worth it, aren't you?

- Select one of these methods: application, inhaler, or mist spray; and use a formula.

- Do the relaxation exercise on page 27. Allow yourself to reach a peaceful, quiet state. Then think about the things you enjoy doing that bring great satisfaction, make you feel good about yourself, and at the same time are beneficial for your well-being.

- Reflect on the *Loving Yourself* affirmation on page 25.

- Repeat this exercise as often as possible. Each session should be about 20 to 30 minutes.

Loving Yourself—Application

Apply one of these formulas to the wrists, upper chest, and back of the neck, until the oil has been fully absorbed into the skin. Bring your wrists close to your nose and breathe the vapors in deeply. When done, if you wish, dab on cornstarch to dry off any remaining oil.

Orange	3 drops
Bergamot	3 drops
Rosewood	2 drops
Helichrysum	2 drops
Carrier Oil	2 teaspoons (10 ml)

Litsea Cubeba	4 drops
Bergamot	2 drops
Chamomile (Roman)	2 drops
Sandalwood	2 drops
Carrier Oil	2 teaspoons (10 ml)

Petitgrain	3 drops
Neroli	3 drops
Chamomile (Roman)	2 drops
Tangerine	2 drops
Carrier Oil	2 teaspoons (10 ml)

Rosewood	3 drops
Chamomile (Roman)	3 drops
Sandalwood	2 drops
Cinnamon Leaf	2 drops
Carrier Oil	2 teaspoons (10 ml)

Helichrysum	4 drops
Cinnamon Leaf	3 drops
Vanilla (CO_2)	3 drops
Carrier Oil	2 teaspoons (10 ml)

Tangerine	4 drops
Sandalwood	3 drops
Vanilla (CO_2)	3 drops
Carrier Oil	2 teaspoons (10 ml)

Litsea Cubeba	4 drops
Mandarin	3 drops
Helichrysum	2 drops
Cinnamon Leaf	1 drop
Carrier Oil	2 teaspoons (10 ml)

Chamomile (Roman)	4 drops
Sandalwood	3 drops
Vanilla (CO_2)	3 drops
Carrier Oil	2 teaspoons (10 ml)

Loving Yourself—Inhaler

Choose one of these formulas. Combine the essential oils in a small glass bottle with a wide opening. Inhale the vapors slowly and deeply. Then tightly cap the bottle after using.

Mandarin	15 drops
Neroli	10 drops
Sandalwood	10 drops

Litsea Cubeba	15 drops
Neroli	10 drops
Rosewood	10 drops

Helichrysum	20 drops
Vanilla (CO_2)	10 drops

Tangerine	15 drops
Litsea Cubeba	10 drops
Cinnamon Leaf	5 drops

Chamomile (Roman)	15 drops
Bergamot	10 drops
Neroli	10 drops

Helichrysum	15 drops
Neroli	10 drops
Spearmint	10 drops

Loving Yourself—Mist Spray

Choose one of these formulas. Fill a fine-mist spray bottle with 2 ounces (60 ml) of purified water, add the essential oils, tighten the cap, and shake well. Mist numerous times over the head with eyes closed. Breathe the vapors in slowly and deeply.

Mandarin	20 drops
Rosewood	20 drops
Geranium	20 drops
Cabreuva	10 drops
Lemongrass	5 drops
Pure Water	2 ounces (60 ml)

Lemon	20 drops
Orange	20 drops
Cardamom	15 drops
Palmarosa	15 drops
Vanilla (CO_2)	5 drops
Pure Water	2 ounces (60 ml)

Grapefruit	15 drops
Geranium	15 drops
Orange	15 drops
Amyris	15 drops
Spearmint	10 drops
Ginger	5 drops
Pure Water	2 ounces (60 ml)

Mandarin	18 drops
Spearmint	17 drops
Rosewood	16 drops
Litsea Cubeba	16 drops
Cinnamon Leaf	8 drops
Pure Water	2 ounces (60 ml)

Orange	26 drops
Litsea Cubeba	25 drops
Vanilla (CO_2)	12 drops
Clove Bud	6 drops
Amyris	6 drops
Pure Water	2 ounces (60 ml)

Tangerine	26 drops
Palmarosa	19 drops
Champaca Flower	10 drops
Amyris	10 drops
Clove Bud	10 drops
Pure Water	2 ounces (60 ml)

Champaca Flower	30 drops
Orange	30 drops
Rosewood	15 drops
Pure Water	2 ounces (60 ml)

Palmarosa	25 drops
Ylang-Ylang	15 drops
Lemon	10 drops
Clove Bud	10 drops
Litsea Cubeba	10 drops
Spearmint	5 drops
Pure Water	2 ounces (60 ml)

MEDITATION

The meditative state relaxes the body and rejuvenates the mind and nervous system.

- Select one of these methods: application, inhaler, or mist spray; and use a formula.

- Do the relaxation exercise on page 27. Allow yourself to reach a peaceful, quiet state of mind and maintain this level of calmness for about 20 to 30 minutes. Practice as often as you wish.

Meditation—Application

Apply one of these formulas to the wrists, upper chest, and back of the neck, until the oil has been fully absorbed into the skin. Bring your wrists close to your nose and breathe the vapors in deeply. When done, if you wish, dab on cornstarch to dry off any remaining oil.

Mandarin	5 drops
Frankincense	4 drops
Amyris	1 drop
Carrier Oil	2 teaspoons (10 ml)

Chamomile (Roman)	5 drops
Tangerine	5 drops
Carrier Oil	2 teaspoons (10 ml)

Chamomile (Roman)	4 drops
Clary Sage	2 drops
Amyris	2 drops
Vanilla (CO_2)	2 drops
Carrier Oil	2 teaspoons (10 ml)

Spruce	5 drops
Cedarwood (Atlas)	4 drops
Nutmeg	1 drop
Carrier Oil	2 teaspoons (10 ml)

Orange	5 drops
Lime	3 drops
Amyris	2 drops
Carrier Oil	2 teaspoons (10 ml)

Chamomile (Roman)	4 drops
Lime	3 drops
Guaiacwood	3 drops
Carrier Oil	2 teaspoons (10 ml)

Tangerine	5 drops
Guaiacwood	3 drops
Ginger	2 drops
Carrier Oil	2 teaspoons (10 ml)

Lime	5 drops
Amyris	5 drops
Carrier Oil	2 teaspoons (10 ml)

Meditation—Inhaler

Choose one of these formulas. Combine the essential oils in a small glass bottle with a wide opening. Inhale the vapors slowly and deeply. Then tightly cap the bottle after using.

Mandarin	15 drops
Guaiacwood	15 drops

Guaiacwood	20 drops
Litsea Cubeba	5 drops

Mandarin	15 drops
Spikenard	10 drops
Chamomile (Roman)	10 drops

Orange	20 drops
Amyris	10 drops

Frankincense	15 drops
Mandarin	15 drops

Frankincense	15 drops
Spruce	15 drops

Meditation—Mist Spray

Choose one of these formulas. Fill a fine-mist spray bottle with 2 ounces (60 ml) of purified water, add the essential oils, tighten the cap, and shake well. Mist numerous times over the head with eyes closed. Breathe the vapors in slowly and deeply.

Mandarin	25 drops
Cedarwood (Atlas)	20 drops
Spruce	20 drops
Litsea Cubeba	10 drops
Pure Water	2 ounces (60 ml)

Chamomile (Roman)	20 drops
Orange	20 drops
Amyris	20 drops
Petitgrain	15 drops
Pure Water	2 ounces (60 ml)

Chamomile (Roman)	25 drops
Tangerine	20 drops
Myrtle	15 drops
Amyris	15 drops
Pure Water	2 ounces (60 ml)

Spruce	30 drops
Frankincense	20 drops
Lemon	15 drops
Cedarwood (Atlas)	10 drops
Pure Water	2 ounces (60 ml)

MENTAL CONCENTRATION

With the advent of high-tech devices, people seem to depend more on machines to do their figuring than on their own minds. These formulas help promote the concentration needed for developing new thoughts and ideas, for planning, creativity, and problem solving. The *Mental Concentration* blends can be valuable when used in conjunction with the input derived from the *Intuition* exercises on page 44.

- Select one of these methods: application, inhaler, or mist spray; and use a formula.

- Spend about 20 to 30 minutes in a quiet, comfortable place and allow yourself to reach a peaceful state. Then write down on a sheet of paper, the thoughts and ideas you came up with and how you will implement them.

- Repeat this exercise as often as possible.

Mental Concentration—Application

Apply one of these formulas to the wrists, upper chest, and back of the neck, until the oil has been fully absorbed into the skin. Bring your wrists close to your nose and breathe the vapors in deeply. When done, if you wish, dab on cornstarch to dry off any remaining oil.

Tangerine	3 drops
Peppermint	3 drops
Cabreuva	2 drops
Cedarwood (Atlas)	2 drops
Carrier Oil	2 teaspoons (10 ml)

Cabreuva	4 drops
Fir Needles	2 drops
Litsea Cubeba	2 drops
Spruce	2 drops
Carrier Oil	2 teaspoons (10 ml)

Ravensara Aromatica	3 drops
Litsea Cubeba	3 drops
Spearmint	3 drops
Helichrysum	1 drop
Carrier Oil	2 teaspoons (10 ml)

Helichrysum	3 drops
Clove Bud	3 drops
Lime	2 drops
Rosemary	2 drops
Carrier Oil	2 teaspoons (10 ml)

Lemon	2 drops
Grapefruit	2 drops
Peppermint	2 drops
Tangerine	2 drops
Rosemary	2 drops
Carrier Oil	2 teaspoons (10 ml)

Cabreuva	2 drops
Spearmint	2 drops
Spruce	2 drops
Lemon	2 drops
Tangerine	2 drops
Carrier Oil	2 teaspoons (10 ml)

Spearmint	4 drops
Tangerine	3 drops
Rosemary	3 drops
Carrier Oil	2 teaspoons (10 ml)

Tangerine	3 drops
Grapefruit	3 drops
Spearmint	3 drops
Cedarwood (Atlas)	1 drop
Carrier Oil	2 teaspoons (10 ml)

Mental Concentration—Inhaler

Choose one of these formulas. Combine the essential oils in a small glass bottle with a wide opening. Inhale the vapors slowly and deeply. Then tightly cap the bottle after using.

Peppermint	25 drops
Cedarwood (Atlas)	10 drops

Eucalyptus Radiata	10 drops
Litsea Cubeba	10 drops
Spearmint	10 drops
Patchouli	5 drops

Litsea Cubeba	15 drops
Peppermint	15 drops
Rosemary	10 drops

Spearmint	15 drops
Spruce	10 drops
Eucalyptus Radiata	10 drops

Peppermint	15 drops
Fir Needles	10 drops
Cedarwood (Atlas)	5 drops

Eucalyptus Radiata	10 drops
Clove Bud	10 drops
Litsea Cubeba	10 drops

Mental Concentration—Mist Spray

Choose one of these formulas. Fill a fine-mist spray bottle with 2 ounces (60 ml) of purified water, add the essential oils, tighten the cap, and shake well. Mist numerous times over the head with eyes closed. Breathe the vapors in slowly and deeply.

Spruce	30 drops
Spearmint	25 drops
Myrtle	10 drops
Lemon	10 drops
Pure Water	2 ounces (60 ml)

Peppermint	25 drops
Eucalyptus Radiata	25 drops
Lemon	25 drops
Pure Water	2 ounces (60 ml)

Spearmint	25 drops
Tangerine	20 drops
Lemon	20 drops
Cedarwood (Atlas)	10 drops
Pure Water	2 ounces (60 ml)

Grapefruit	20 drops
Basil (Sweet)	20 drops
Spearmint	20 drops
Litsea Cubeba	15 drops
Pure Water	2 ounces (60 ml)

Eucalyptus Citriodora	20 drops
Lemon	20 drops
Tangerine	18 drops
Cabreuva	17 drops
Pure Water	2 ounces (60 ml)

Lemon	25 drops
Ravensara Aromatica	20 drops
Spearmint	20 drops
Cedarwood (Atlas)	10 drops
Pure Water	2 ounces (60 ml)

Lemon	23 drops
Tangerine	22 drops
Basil (Sweet)	15 drops
Spruce	15 drops
Pure Water	2 ounces (60 ml)

Spruce	25 drops
Spearmint	18 drops
Tangerine	17 drops
Clove Bud	15 drops
Pure Water	2 ounces (60 ml)

Litsea Cubeba	28 drops
Spearmint	27 drops
Rosemary	15 drops
Cedarwood (Atlas)	5 drops
Pure Water	2 ounces (60 ml)

Tangerine	30 drops
Hyssop Decumbens	15 drops
Cedarwood (Atlas)	10 drops
Spruce	10 drops
Clove Bud	10 drops
Pure Water	2 ounces (60 ml)

Cajeput	25 drops
Peppermint	25 drops
Lime	25 drops
Pure Water	2 ounces (60 ml)

Lime	30 drops
Peppermint	20 drops
Rosemary	15 drops
Cardamom	10 drops
Pure Water	2 ounces (60 ml)

MOTIVATION

- Select one of these methods: application, inhaler, or mist spray; and use a formula.

- Do the relaxation exercise on page 27. Allow yourself to reach a peaceful, quiet state of mind. Then reflect on the things you are motivated to do that are beneficial to yourself and others, for the highest good. Write down on a sheet of paper what they are and the actions you are going to take. A few examples are being motivated at work to serve your customers to the best of your ability, creating a good habit like improving your self-discipline, or reading books on how to prepare healthier meals for yourself and your loved ones.

- Repeat this exercise as often as possible. Each session should be about 20 to 30 minutes.

Motivation—Application

Apply one of these formulas to the wrists, upper chest, and back of the neck, until the oil has been fully absorbed into the skin. Bring your wrists close to your nose and breathe the vapors in deeply. When done, if you wish, dab on cornstarch to dry off any remaining oil.

Helichrysum	4 drops
Neroli	2 drops
Peppermint	2 drops
Patchouli	2 drops
Carrier Oil	2 teaspoons (10 ml)

Litsea Cubeba	3 drops
Mandarin	3 drops
Vanilla (CO_2)	2 drops
Peppermint	2 drops
Carrier Oil	2 teaspoons (10 ml)

Spearmint	3 drops
Mandarin	3 drops
Helichrysum	2 drops
Vanilla (CO_2)	2 drops
Carrier Oil	2 teaspoons (10 ml)

Spearmint	3 drops
Litsea Cubeba	3 drops
Patchouli	2 drops
Helichrysum	2 drops
Carrier Oil	2 teaspoons (10 ml)

Rosewood	2 drops
Cardamom	2 drops
Mandarin	2 drops
Bergamot	2 drops
Helichrysum	2 drops
Carrier Oil	2 teaspoons (10 ml)

Litsea Cubeba	4 drops
Patchouli	2 drops
Vanilla (CO_2)	2 drops
Tangerine	2 drops
Carrier Oil	2 teaspoons (10 ml)

Spearmint	3 drops
Litsea Cubeba	3 drops
Patchouli	2 drops
Vanilla (CO_2)	1 drop
Rosemary	1 drop
Carrier Oil	2 teaspoons (10 ml)

Spearmint	3 drops
Mandarin	3 drops
Amyris	2 drops
Rose	2 drops
Carrier Oil	2 teaspoons (10 ml)

Lemon	3 drops
Vanilla (CO_2)	3 drop
Fennel (Sweet)	2 drops
Patchouli	2 drops
Carrier Oil	2 teaspoons (10 ml)

Amyris	2 drops
Eucalyptus Radiata	2 drops
Peppermint	2 drops
Orange	2 drops
Cardamom	2 drops
Carrier Oil	2 teaspoons (10 ml)

Motivation—Inhaler

Choose one of these formulas. Combine the essential oils in a small glass bottle with a wide opening. Inhale the vapors slowly and deeply. Then tightly cap the bottle after using.

Spearmint	15 drops
Tangerine	10 drops
Clove Bud	5 drops
Litsea Cubeba	5 drops

Grapefruit	10 drops
Eucalyptus Radiata	10 drops
Litsea Cubeba	10 drops
Patchouli	5 drops

Rosewood	20 drops
Tangerine	15 drops

Spearmint	20 drops
Orange	10 drops
Amyris	5 drops

Litsea Cubeba	25 drops
Tangerine	25 drops
Helichrysum	10 drops
Amyris	10 drops
Cardamom	5 drops
Pure Water	2 ounces (60 ml)

Lemon	30 drops
Peppermint	25 drops
Litsea Cubeba	15 drops
Patchouli	5 drops
Pure Water	2 ounces (60 ml)

MOTIVES FOR OUR ACTIONS

This exercise can be a valuable means of understanding how honest we are with ourselves. It can help us lessen inner conflicts and eventually create a state of inner peacefulness and well-being.

- Select one of these methods: application, inhaler, or mist spray; and use a formula.

- Do the relaxation exercise on page 27. Allow yourself to reach a peaceful, quiet state of mind. Then write down on a sheet of paper, the actions you take and the motives behind them. Examine each one and determine how sincere your intentions are and if you can improve on them.

- Repeat this exercise as often as possible. Each session should be about 20 to 30 minutes.

Motives for Our Actions—Application

Apply one of these formulas to the wrists, upper chest, and back of the neck, until the oil has been fully absorbed into the skin. Bring your wrists close to your nose and breathe the vapors in deeply. When done, if you wish, dab on cornstarch to dry off any remaining oil.

Motivation—Mist Spray

Choose one of these formulas. Fill a fine-mist spray bottle with 2 ounces (60 ml) of purified water, add the essential oils, tighten the cap, and shake well. Mist numerous times over the head with eyes closed. Breathe the vapors in slowly and deeply.

Spearmint	25 drops
Litsea Cubeba	25 drops
Mandarin	19 drops
Vanilla (CO_2)	6 drops
Pure Water	2 ounces (60 ml)

Tangerine	30 drops
Spearmint	25 drops
Eucalyptus Radiata	10 drops
Fennel (Sweet)	5 drops
Amyris	5 drops
Pure Water	2 ounces (60 ml)

Spruce	4 drops
Frankincense	3 drops
Litsea Cubeba	3 drops
Carrier Oil	2 teaspoons (10 ml)

Chamomile (Roman)	4 drops
Dill	3 drops
Amyris	3 drops
Carrier Oil	2 teaspoons (10 ml)

Fir Needles	4 drops
Spruce	3 drops
Spikenard	3 drops
Carrier Oil	2 teaspoons (10 ml)

Rosewood	4 drops
Tangerine	4 drops
Sage (Spanish)	2 drops
Carrier Oil	2 teaspoons (10 ml)

Frankincense	4 drops
Lime	4 drops
Cedarwood (Atlas)	2 drops
Carrier Oil	2 teaspoons (10 ml)

Spruce	4 drops
Galbanum	3 drops
Vanilla (CO_2)	3 drops
Carrier Oil	2 teaspoons (10 ml)

Lemon	4 drops
Spikenard	3 drops
Spruce	3 drops
Carrier Oil	2 teaspoons (10 ml)

Spruce	5 drops
Amyris	5 drops
Carrier Oil	2 teaspoons (10 ml)

Motives for Our Actions—Inhaler

Choose one of these formulas. Combine the essential oils in a small glass bottle with a wide opening. Inhale the vapors slowly and deeply. Then tightly cap the bottle after using.

Spruce	10 drops
Tangerine	10 drops
Guaiacwood	10 drops

Chamomile (Roman)	15 drops
Vanilla (CO_2)	5 drops

Spruce	15 drops
Fir Needles	10 drops
Spikenard	10 drops

Tangerine	10 drops
Dill	10 drops
Neroli	10 drops

Chamomile (Roman)	10 drops
Litsea Cubeba	10 drops
Frankincense	10 drops

Spruce	15 drops
Myrtle	10 drops
Cedarwood (Atlas)	5 drops

Motives for Our Actions—Mist Spray

Choose one of these formulas. Fill a fine-mist spray bottle with 2 ounces (60 ml) of purified water, add the essential oils, tighten the cap, and shake well. Mist numerous times over the head with eyes closed. Breathe the vapors in slowly and deeply.

Rosewood	20 drops
Dill	15 drops
Litsea Cubeba	15 drops
Tangerine	15 drops
Chamomile (Roman)	10 drops
Pure Water	2 ounces (60 ml)

Spruce	20 drops
Fir Needles	20 drops
Petitgrain	20 drops
Cedarwood (Atlas)	15 drops
Pure Water	2 ounces (60 ml)

Fir Needles	25 drops
Lime	20 drops
Myrtle	15 drops
Cedarwood (Atlas)	15 drops
Pure Water	2 ounces (60 ml)

Frankincense	25 drops
Fir Needles	20 drops
Spruce	20 drops
Amyris	10 drops
Pure Water	2 ounces (60 ml)

REFLECTION

The path you have followed in prior years brought you to where you are now. The path you are on now will determine where you will be in future years. Are you presently on the right path to where you want to be?

- Select one of these methods: application, inhaler, or mist spray; and use a formula.

- Do the relaxation exercise on page 27. Allow yourself to reach a peaceful, quiet state. Then reflect on your path. List on a sheet of paper the insights on your direction in life, the changes needed to be on your path, and the actions you have committed to take.

- Repeat this exercise as often as you feel necessary. Each session should be about 20 to 30 minutes.

Reflection—Application

Apply one of these formulas to the wrists, upper chest, and back of the neck, until the oil has been fully absorbed into the skin. Bring your wrists close to your nose and breathe the vapors in deeply. When done, if you wish, dab on cornstarch to dry off any remaining oil.

Chamomile (Roman)	3 drops
Basil (Sweet)	3 drops
Cinnamon Leaf	2 drops
Spikenard	2 drops
Carrier Oil	2 teaspoons (10 ml)

Litsea Cubeba	4 drops
Basil (Sweet)	3 drops
Spikenard	3 drops
Carrier Oil	2 teaspoons (10 ml)

Helichrysum	5 drops
Vetiver	3 drops
Tangerine	2 drops
Carrier Oil	2 teaspoons (10 ml)

Helichrysum	4 drops
Fir Needles	2 drops
Guaiacwood	2 drops
Vanilla (CO_2)	2 drops
Carrier Oil	2 teaspoons (10 ml)

Juniper Berry	4 drops
Spruce	3 drops
Guaiacwood	3 drops
Carrier Oil	2 teaspoons (10 ml)

Helichrysum	3 drops
Basil (Sweet)	3 drops
Cinnamon Leaf	3 drops
Frankincense	1 drop
Carrier Oil	2 teaspoons (10 ml)

Spruce	4 drops
Cedarwood (Atlas)	3 drops
Vanilla (CO_2)	3 drops
Carrier Oil	2 teaspoons (10 ml)

Tangerine	4 drops
Spikenard	4 drops
Vanilla (CO_2)	2 drops
Carrier Oil	2 teaspoons (10 ml)

Reflection—Inhaler

Choose one of these formulas. Combine the essential oils in a small glass bottle with a wide opening. Inhale the vapors slowly and deeply. Then tightly cap the bottle after using.

Helichrysum	20 drops
Spikenard	5 drops

Helichrysum	15 drops
Basil (Sweet)	10 drops
Guaiacwood	10 drops

Spruce	25 drops
Cedarwood (Atlas)	5 drops

Frankincense	20 drops
Cedarwood (Atlas)	5 drops
Lemon	5 drops

Litsea Cubeba	15 drops
Spikenard	5 drops

Fir Needles	20 drops
Cinnamon Leaf	5 drops

Reflection—Mist Spray

Choose one of these formulas. Fill a fine-mist spray bottle with 2 ounces (60 ml) of purified water, add the essential oils, tighten the cap, and shake well. Mist numerous times over the head with eyes closed. Breathe the vapors in slowly and deeply.

Tangerine	20 drops
Helichrysum	20 drops
Myrtle	20 drops
Amyris	15 drops
Pure Water	2 ounces (60 ml)

Litsea Cubeba	25 drops
Juniper Berry	20 drops
Spruce	15 drops
Amyris	15 drops
Pure Water	2 ounces (60 ml)

Spruce	20 drops
Juniper Berry	15 drops
Helichrysum	15 drops
Tangerine	15 drops
Amyris	10 drops
Pure Water	2 ounces (60 ml)

Spruce	20 drops
Fir Needles	20 drops
Basil (Sweet)	15 drops
Cedarwood (Atlas)	10 drops
Lemon	10 drops
Pure Water	2 ounces (60 ml)

RELINQUISH SELFISHNESS

Many people engage in acts of selfishness. For example, siblings fight a bitter battle, each one wanting to get a larger portion of their deceased parents' inheritance. A driver cuts in front of another vehicle to get a parking space. A person sprays pesticide and herbicide in his yard to eliminate weeds and insects. The spray drifts over to his neighbor's property into an organic vegetable garden. His neighbor's food is now contaminated and so is the quality of the air he has to breathe. A pregnant woman doesn't take care of herself properly when she eats a poor diet, thus depriving herself and her unborn child of proper nutrition.

If you have selfish behaviors, these formulas and exercise can help you to realize and overcome them.

- Select one of these methods: application, inhaler or mist spray; and use a formula.

- Do the relaxation exercise on page 27. Allow yourself to reach a peaceful, quiet state. Then ponder the acts you have taken that displayed selfishness. Write down on a sheet of paper, these acts and how you will be more unselfish from now on. Continue practicing this exercise until you make changes and relinquish your selfishness.

- Each session should be about 20 to 30 minutes.

Relinquish Selfishness—Application

Apply one of these formulas to the wrists, upper chest, abdomen, and back of the neck, until the oil has been fully absorbed into the skin. Bring your wrists close to your nose and breathe the vapors in deeply. When done, if you wish, dab on cornstarch to dry off any remaining oil.

Vanilla (CO_2)	4 drops
Tangerine	2 drops
Neroli	2 drops
Amyris	2 drops
Carrier Oil	2 teaspoons (10 ml)

Citronella	3 drops
Mandarin	3 drops
Vanilla (CO_2)	2 drops
Cedarwood (Atlas)	2 drops
Carrier Oil	2 teaspoons (10 ml)

Cardamom	3 drops
Palmarosa	3 drops
Vanilla (CO_2)	2 drops
Tangerine	2 drops
Carrier Oil	2 teaspoons (10 ml)

Helichrysum	3 drops
Clary Sage	3 drops
Lemon	2 drops
Guaiacwood	2 drops
Carrier Oil	2 teaspoons (10 ml)

Chamomile (Roman)	3 drops
Citronella	3 drops
Galbanum	2 drops
Vanilla (CO_2)	2 drops
Carrier Oil	2 teaspoons (10 ml)

Vanilla (CO_2)	3 drops
Cinnamon Leaf	3 drops
Spruce	2 drops
Helichrysum	2 drops
Carrier Oil	2 teaspoons (10 ml)

Lemon	3 drops
Frankincense	3 drops
Cardamom	2 drops
Palmarosa	2 drops
Carrier Oil	2 teaspoons (10 ml)

Galbanum	3 drops
Neroli	3 drops
Litsea Cubeba	2 drops
Amyris	2 drops
Carrier Oil	2 teaspoons (10 ml)

Chamomile (Roman)	3 drops
Vanilla (CO_2)	3 drops
Citronella	2 drops
Dill	2 drops
Carrier Oil	2 teaspoons (10 ml)

Tangerine	3 drops
Anise	2 drops
Chamomile (Roman)	2 drops
Citronella	2 drops
Nutmeg	1 drop
Carrier Oil	2 teaspoons (10 ml)

Relinquish Selfishness—Inhaler

Choose one of these formulas. Combine the essential oils in a small glass bottle with a wide opening. Inhale the vapors slowly and deeply. Then tightly cap the bottle after using.

Citronella	15 drops
Vanilla (CO_2)	7 drops

Spruce	10 drops
Vanilla (CO_2)	5 drops

Tangerine	10 drops
Frankincense	5 drops
Cedarwood (Atlas)	5 drops

Chamomile (Roman)	10 drops
Champaca Flower	5 drops

Relinquish Selfishness—Mist Spray

Choose one of these formulas. Fill a fine-mist spray bottle with 2 ounces (60 ml) of purified water, add the essential oils, tighten the cap, and shake well. Mist numerous times over the head with eyes closed. Breathe the vapors in slowly and deeply.

Tangerine	25 drops
Citronella	20 drops
Copaiba	15 drops
Fennel (Sweet)	15 drops
Pure Water	2 ounces (60 ml)

Spruce	30 drops
Lemon	20 drops
Clove Bud	10 drops
Spearmint	10 drops
Guaiacwood	5 drops
Pure Water	2 ounces (60 ml)

Spruce	25 drops
Fir Needles	25 drops
Litsea Cubeba	13 drops
Fennel (Sweet)	12 drops
Pure Water	2 ounces (60 ml)

Chamomile (Roman)	20 drops
Citronella	15 drops
Spruce	15 drops
Vanilla (CO_2)	15 drops
Copaiba	10 drops
Pure Water	2 ounces (60 ml)

Lemon	25 drops
Tangerine	25 drops
Neroli	15 drops
Sage (Spanish)	10 drops
Pure Water	2 ounces (60 ml)

Citronella	30 drops
Tangerine	15 drops
Sage (Spanish)	15 drops
Cedarwood (Atlas)	15 drops
Pure Water	2 ounces (60 ml)

THINK POSITIVE THOUGHTS

We are today a product of our past thoughts, which influenced us to make the decisions we made and led us to take the actions we took. The same holds true now. The thoughts we have today will determine the decisions and actions that will shape our life in future years. It is important for us to promote positive thoughts to help brighten our outlook for the years ahead.

- Select one of these methods: application, inhaler or mist spray; and use a formula.

- Do the relaxation exercise on page 27. Allow yourself to be surrounded with positive energy. Think of the positive actions you need to take to improve your life. Record your thoughts on a sheet of paper. List specific situations that you are in that you may be able to improve by thinking and acting more positively. Write the positive thoughts for each situation and the positive actions to take. Place this sheet where it is easily visible so that you can often refer to it. After three months of taking action, write the results and benefits of doing this exercise.

- Repeat this exercise three times for the first week, then as often as you feel necessary. Each session should be about 20 to 30 minutes.

Think Positive Thoughts—Application

Apply one of these formulas to the wrists, upper chest, and back of the neck, until the oil has been fully absorbed into the skin. Bring your wrists close to your nose and breathe the vapors in deeply. When done, if you wish, dab on cornstarch to dry off any remaining oil.

Spearmint	4 drops
Helichrysum	3 drops
Sandalwood	3 drops
Carrier Oil	2 teaspoons (10 ml)

Spruce	4 drops
Litsea Cubeba	4 drops
Vanilla (CO_2)	2 drops
Carrier Oil	2 teaspoons (10 ml)

Petitgrain	3 drops
Lemon	3 drops
Neroli	3 drops
Cedarwood (Atlas)	1 drop
Carrier Oil	2 teaspoons (10 ml)

Tangerine	4 drops
Petitgrain	3 drops
Champaca Flower	3 drops
Carrier Oil	2 teaspoons (10 ml)

Think Positive Thoughts—Inhaler

Choose one of these formulas. Combine the essential oils in a small glass bottle with a wide opening. Inhale the vapors slowly and deeply. Then tightly cap the bottle after using.

Orange	20 drops
Helichrysum	10 drops

Petitgrain	10 drops
Neroli	10 drops

Spruce	15 drops
Tangerine	15 drops

Peppermint	20 drops
Spikenard	5 drops

Think Positive Thoughts—Mist Spray

Choose one of these formulas. Fill a fine-mist spray bottle with 2 ounces (60 ml) of purified water, add the essential oils, tighten the cap, and shake well. Mist numerous times over the head with eyes closed. Breathe the vapors in slowly and deeply.

Helichrysum	25 drops
Champaca Flower	20 drops
Citronella	20 drops
Cedarwood (Atlas)	10 drops
Pure Water	2 ounces (60 ml)

Spruce	22 drops
Spearmint	18 drops
Thyme	18 drops
Amyris	17 drops
Pure Water	2 ounces (60 ml)

Tangerine	30 drops
Cedarwood (Atlas)	20 drops
Dill	15 drops
Neroli	10 drops
Pure Water	2 ounces (60 ml)

Copaiba	20 drops
Orange	20 drops
Cardamom	20 drops
Helichrysum	15 drops
Pure Water	2 ounces (60 ml)

VISUALIZATION

Visualization is helpful to accomplish a goal. Repeatedly going over every step in picture form in the mind helps make the goal more real.

- Select one of these methods: application, inhaler, or mist spray; and use a formula.

- Do the relaxation exercise on page 27. Allow yourself to reach a peaceful, quiet state. Then write down on a sheet of paper, in detail what you want to see yourself accomplish. Afterwards, envision yourself in every detail from beginning to end accomplishing the desired goal. An example of a goal can be mastering one or more of the twenty-two virtues of higher consciousness. See yourself successful. After doing the visualization exercise, make a note on the paper of the experience, so that you will have it to refer back to next time.

If doubts, contradictory thoughts, or negative feelings present themselves during or after the visualization, allow them to pass. Don't analyze, suppress, or resist them, since resistance gives them power by diverting your thoughts. Just return to your positive vision, and the doubts and negative feelings will leave of their own accord.

- Repeat this exercise as often as possible, ideally three to four times a week for about 20 to 30 minutes each time. The more you practice the visualization, the easier it will become.

Visualization—Application

Apply one of these formulas to the wrists, upper chest, and back of the neck, until the oil has been fully absorbed into the skin. Bring your wrists close to your nose and breathe the vapors in deeply. When done, if you wish, dab on cornstarch to dry off any remaining oil.

Helichrysum	5 drops
Basil (Sweet)	3 drops
Cinnamon Leaf	2 drops
Carrier Oil	2 teaspoons (10 ml)

Lemon	4 drops
Clary Sage	3 drops
Basil (Sweet)	3 drops
Carrier Oil	2 teaspoons (10 ml)

Chamomile (Roman)	4 drops
Basil (Sweet)	2 drops
Vanilla (CO_2)	2 drops
Lavender	2 drops
Carrier Oil	2 teaspoons (10 ml)

Frankincense	4 drops
Juniper Berry	3 drops
Cinnamon Leaf	3 drops
Carrier Oil	2 teaspoons (10 ml)

Frankincense	4 drops
Tangerine	2 drops
Lemon	2 drops
Cinnamon Leaf	2 drops
Carrier Oil	2 teaspoons (10 ml)

Chamomile (Roman)	4 drops
Tangerine	3 drops
Clary Sage	3 drops
Carrier Oil	2 teaspoons (10 ml)

Visualization—Inhaler

Choose one of these formulas. Combine the essential oils in a small glass bottle with a wide opening. Inhale the vapors slowly and deeply. Then tightly cap the bottle after using.

| Frankincense | 15 drops |
| Spruce | 15 drops |

Frankincense	10 drops
Helichrysum	10 drops
Lavender	10 drops

| Chamomile (Roman) | 15 drops |
| Clary Sage | 10 drops |

Helichrysum	10 drops
Basil (Sweet)	10 drops
Cedarwood (Atlas)	10 drops

Visualization—Mist Spray

Choose one of these formulas. Fill a fine-mist spray bottle with 2 ounces (60 ml) of purified water, add the essential oils, tighten the cap, and shake well. Mist numerous times over the head with eyes closed. Breathe the vapors in slowly and deeply.

Spruce	35 drops
Basil (Sweet)	15 drops
Helichrysum	15 drops
Mandarin	10 drops
Pure Water	2 ounces (60 ml)

Mandarin	30 drops
Petitgrain	15 drops
Lemon	15 drops
Basil (Sweet)	10 drops
Cedarwood (Atlas)	5 drops
Pure Water	2 ounces (60 ml)

Tangerine	20 drops
Lemon	20 drops
Spruce	20 drops
Amyris	15 drops
Pure Water	2 ounces (60 ml)

Chamomile (Roman)	25 drops
Tangerine	20 drops
Lemon	20 drops
Cedarwood (Atlas)	10 drops
Pure Water	2 ounces (60 ml)

CHAPTER 5

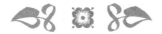

Enjoying Life More

The power that created us wants us to have a great life, and we owe it to ourselves to do so.

We are often faced with so many demands, responsibilities, and obligations that sometimes we lose ourselves in the midst of trying to keep up. Life is too short to let the days rush by without experiencing the simple pleasures that are so worthwhile and beautiful. So set aside time today to enjoy nature; start everyday off with the *Morning Affirmation* (page 81); and do the other exercises to attain a more fulfilled, meaningful life that you are meant to have. Don't let another day pass without enjoying life to the fullest.

BE THE BEST YOU CAN BE

It is unfortunate that there are people who possess phenomenal skills, talents, and valuable knowledge but make little or no use of these great attributes. It is so important to utilize all that we have, to make a better and more meaningful life for ourselves and the people we care for—and to develop into nothing less than our fullest potential.

- Select one of these methods: application, diffuser, inhaler, or mist spray; and choose a formula.

- Find a quiet, comfortable place to relax where you will not be disturbed, play soft music (optional), and use the formula. Close your eyes and spend about 20 to 30 minutes pondering the skills, talents, and knowledge you possess that you haven't been utilizing to the fullest. Then list them on a sheet of paper. Write an action plan that will keep you focused to be the best you can be and reach your full potential. After every week, measure the progress you've made and make adjustments to your action plan if necessary.

- Repeat this exercise until optimal results are obtained.

Be the Best You Can Be—Application

Apply one of these formulas to the wrists, upper chest, and back of the neck, until the oil has been fully absorbed into the skin. Bring your wrists close to your nose and breathe the vapors in deeply. When done, if you wish, dab on cornstarch to dry off any remaining oil.

Tangerine	3 drops
Litsea Cubeba	3 drops
Patchouli	2 drops
Neroli	2 drops
Carrier Oil	2 teaspoons (10 ml)

Guaiacwood	4 drops
Litsea Cubeba	2 drops
Orange	2 drops
Spearmint	2 drops
Carrier Oil	2 teaspoons (10 ml)

Litsea Cubeba	4 drops
Helichrysum	2 drops
Cinnamon Leaf	2 drops
Rose	2 drops
Carrier Oil	2 teaspoons (10 ml)

Sandalwood	3 drops
Basil (Sweet)	3 drops
Allspice Berry	2 drops
Rose	2 drops
Carrier Oil	2 teaspoons (10 ml)

Spruce	4 drops
Neroli	3 drops
Tangerine	3 drops
Carrier Oil	2 teaspoons (10 ml)

Vanilla (CO_2)	4 drops
Fennel (Sweet)	3 drops
Allspice Berry	3 drops
Carrier Oil	2 teaspoons (10 ml)

Be the Best You Can Be—Diffuser

Choose one of these formulas. Depending on the type of diffuser you have, place the essential oils in the designated area, then turn on the unit to disperse the aroma into the air.

Orange	40%
Grapefruit	30%
Litsea Cubeba	20%
Allspice Berry	10%

| Spruce | 50% |
| Lemon | 50% |

| Spearmint | 50% |
| Orange | 50% |

| Spruce | 50% |
| Spearmint | 50% |

Be the Best You Can Be—Inhaler

Choose one of these formulas. Combine the essential oils in a small glass bottle with a wide opening. Inhale the vapors slowly and deeply. Then tightly cap the bottle after using.

| Orange | 30 drops |
| Rose | 5 drops |

Orange	20 drops
Vanilla (CO_2)	5 drops
Spearmint	5 drops

Orange	20 drops
Litsea Cubeba	10 drops
Patchouli	5 drops

Bergamot	15 drops
Spearmint	10 drops
Patchouli	5 drops

Be the Best You Can Be—Mist Spray

Choose one of these formulas. Fill a fine-mist spray bottle with 2 ounces (60 ml) of purified water, add the essential oils, tighten the cap, and shake well. Mist numerous times over the head with eyes closed. Breathe the vapors in slowly and deeply.

Orange	25 drops
Lemon	25 drops
Cedarwood (Atlas)	17 drops
Rosewood	8 drops
Pure Water	2 ounces (60 ml)

Tangerine	20 drops
Grapefruit	20 drops
Litsea Cubeba	20 drops
Allspice Berry	10 drops
Patchouli	5 drops
Pure Water	2 ounces (60 ml)

Lemon	25 drops
Orange	20 drops
Spearmint	20 drops
Patchouli	10 drops
Pure Water	2 ounces (60 ml)

Spruce	20 drops
Spearmint	20 drops
Basil (Sweet)	15 drops
Tangerine	15 drops
Vanilla (CO_2)	5 drops
Pure Water	2 ounces (60 ml)

CHOOSE TO BE HAPPY

Some people seemingly have everything going for them—good looks, personality, intelligence, and talent—but yet they are not happy, while other people can make themselves happy with very little. Long-term happiness comes from deep within. It is a mind-set, an attitude reflecting our perceptions and the things we do to derive satisfaction out of life. Once you've decided that you want to be happy, these formulas can enhance your mood.

- Select one of these methods: application, inhaler, or mist spray; and choose a formula.

- Find a quiet, comfortable place to relax where you will not be disturbed, play soft music (optional), and use the formula. Close your eyes and spend about 20 to 30 minutes reflecting on improving your attitude and perceptions to get more satisfaction out of your life.

- Reflect on the *Loving Yourself* affirmation on page 25.

Choose to Be Happy—Application

Apply one of these formulas to the wrists, upper chest, and back of the neck, until the oil has been fully absorbed into the skin. Bring your wrists close to your nose and breathe the vapors in deeply. When done, if you wish, dab on cornstarch to dry off any remaining oil.

Champaca Flower	3 drops
Vanilla (CO_2)	3 drops
Litsea Cubeba	3 drops
Patchouli	1 drop
Carrier Oil	2 teaspoons (10 ml)

Tangerine	4 drops
Rose	2 drops
Champaca Flower	2 drops
Allspice Berry	2 drops
Carrier Oil	2 teaspoons (10 ml)

Spearmint	3 drops
Sandalwood	3 drops
Hyssop Decumbens	2 drops
Neroli	2 drops
Carrier Oil	2 teaspoons (10 ml)

Lemon	3 drops
Ylang-Ylang	3 drops
Champaca Flower	2 drops
Neroli	2 drops
Carrier Oil	2 teaspoons (10 ml)

Helichrysum	2 drops
Neroli	2 drops
Ylang-Ylang	2 drops
Grapefruit	2 drops
Palmarosa	2 drops
Carrier Oil	2 teaspoons (10 ml)

Geranium	2 drops
Mandarin	2 drops
Lemon Myrtle	2 drops
Rosewood	2 drops
Spikenard	2 drops
Carrier Oil	2 teaspoons (10 ml)

Choose to Be Happy—Inhaler

Choose one of these formulas. Combine the essential oils in a small glass bottle with a wide opening. Inhale the vapors slowly and deeply. Then tightly cap the bottle after using.

Mandarin	20 drops
Litsea Cubeba	5 drops
Vanilla (CO_2)	2 drops

Orange	20 drops
Spearmint	10 drops
Spikenard	5 drops

Spearmint	20 drops
Vanilla (CO_2)	5 drops

Litsea Cubeba	10 drops
Ylang-Ylang	10 drops

Choose to Be Happy—Mist Spray

Choose one of these formulas. Fill a fine-mist spray bottle with 2 ounces (60 ml) of purified water, add the essential oils, tighten the cap, and

shake well. Mist numerous times over the head with eyes closed. Breathe the vapors in slowly and deeply.

Spearmint	30 drops
Clove Bud	18 drops
Litsea Cubeba	17 drops
Patchouli	10 drops
Pure Water	2 ounces (60 ml)

Mandarin	25 drops
Cardamom	20 drops
Lemon	15 drops
Spearmint	15 drops
Pure Water	2 ounces (60 ml)

Bergamot	30 drops
Ylang-Ylang	20 drops
Grapefruit	15 drops
Vetiver	10 drops
Pure Water	2 ounces (60 ml)

Lemon	20 drops
Tangerine	20 drops
Copaiba	13 drops
Clove Bud	12 drops
Helichrysum	10 drops
Pure Water	2 ounces (60 ml)

COMMUNICATE EFFECTIVELY

Proper communication is a great tool to prevent or solve problems and disagreements between people. But there are times when we are extremely hurt or offended due to what someone has done to us. At that point, our communication may turn into an attack instrument to hurt the other individual. When in such a situation, use one of these formulas to relax and help dissipate the hurt.

- Select one of these methods: application, inhaler, or mist spray; and choose a formula.

- Find a quiet, comfortable place to relax where you will not be disturbed, play soft music (optional), and use the formula. Spend about 20 to 30 minutes and write down on a sheet of paper why you feel angry or hurt. Then, write what you want to say in a polite and most effective way to minimize the conflict and make peace, either with the person and/or within yourself.

- Depending on the depth of anger or hurt, you may need to practice this exercise several times to obtain best results.

Communicate Effectively—Application

Apply one of these formulas to the wrists, upper chest, and back of the neck, until the oil has been fully absorbed into the skin. Bring your wrists close to your nose and breathe the vapors in deeply. When done, if you wish, dab on cornstarch to dry off any remaining oil.

Spruce	4 drops
Lime	3 drops
Copaiba	3 drops
Carrier Oil	2 teaspoons (10 ml)

Lime	4 drops
Chamomile (Roman)	2 drops
Vanilla (CO_2)	2 drops
Spearmint	2 drops
Carrier Oil	2 teaspoons (10 ml)

Chamomile (Roman)	3 drops
Tangerine	3 drops
Vanilla (CO_2)	2 drops
Peppermint	2 drops
Carrier Oil	2 teaspoons (10 ml)

Geranium	3 drops
Fennel (Sweet)	2 drops
Vanilla (CO_2)	2 drops
Allspice Berry	2 drops
Spearmint	1 drop
Carrier Oil	2 teaspoons (10 ml)

Cedarwood (Atlas)	4 drops
Spruce	4 drops
Litsea Cubeba	2 drops
Carrier Oil	2 teaspoons (10 ml)

Spruce	4 drops
Lemon	3 drops
Chamomile (Roman)	3 drops
Carrier Oil	2 teaspoons (10 ml)

Helichrysum	4 drops
Peppermint	3 drops
Cadarmom	3 drops
Carrier Oil	2 teaspoons (10 ml)

Spearmint	5 drops
Lemon	3 drops
Basil (Sweet)	2 drops
Carrier Oil	2 teaspoons (10 ml)

Communicate Effectively—Inhaler

Choose one of these formulas. Combine the essential oils in a small glass bottle with a wide opening. Inhale the vapors slowly and deeply. Then tightly cap the bottle after using.

Spearmint	20 drops
Lemon	10 drops

Spearmint	20 drops
Chamomile (Roman)	10 drops

Tangerine	15 drops
Spearmint	10 drops
Litsea Cubeba	5 drops
Chamomile (Roman)	5 drops

Spearmint	15 drops
Tangerine	15 drops

Spruce	15 drops
Eucalyptus Citriodora	10 drops
Lemon	5 drops

Tangerine	17 drops
Spruce	13 drops

Lime	15 drops
Spearmint	15 drops
Amyris	5 drops

Spearmint	23 drops
Orange	5 drops
Anise	3 drops

Communicate Effectively—Mist Spray

Choose one of these formulas. Fill a fine-mist spray bottle with 2 ounces (60 ml) of purified water, add the essential oils, tighten the cap, and shake well. Mist numerous times over the head with eyes closed. Breathe the vapors in slowly and deeply.

Spearmint	25 drops
Orange	25 drops
Cedarwood (Atlas)	25 drops
Pure Water	2 ounces (60 ml)

Spruce	30 drops
Copaiba	25 drops
Tangerine	10 drops
Lemongrass	10 drops
Pure Water	2 ounces (60 ml)

Helichrysum	25 drops
Spearmint	25 drops
Fennel (Sweet)	9 drops
Allspice Berry	8 drops
Lemongrass	8 drops
Pure Water	2 ounces (60 ml)

Spruce	30 drops
Peppermint	30 drops
Chamomile (Roman)	15 drops
Pure Water	2 ounces (60 ml)

Spearmint	35 drops
Spruce	20 drops
Peppermint	10 drops
Lime	10 drops
Pure Water	2 ounces (60 ml)

Spearmint	25 drops
Spruce	15 drops
Helichrysum	13 drops
Clove Bud	12 drops
Vanilla (CO_2)	10 drops
Pure Water	2 ounces (60 ml)

CONFIDENCE FOR A MEETING

Attending events and meetings can be stressful, especially if you have to give a presentation. Use these formulas to reduce stress and help boost self-confidence.

Confidence for a Meeting—Application

Choose one of these formulas. Prior to leaving for the meeting, apply the formula on the wrists, upper chest, back of the neck, and shoulders. Rub in well until the oil is fully absorbed into the skin. Bring your wrists close to your nose and breathe the vapors in deeply. After the application, if you wish, dab on cornstarch to dry off any remaining oil. When you are ready to go to the meeting, you may also want to take the *Confidence for a Meeting* inhaler along with you.

Helichrysum	4 drops
Spearmint	3 drops
Lemon	3 drops
Carrier Oil	2 teaspoons (10 ml)

Lemon	4 drops
Neroli	3 drops
Coriander	3 drops
Carrier Oil	2 teaspoons (10 ml)

Spearmint	4 drops
Vanilla (CO_2)	3 drops
Grapefruit	3 drops
Carrier Oil	2 teaspoons (10 ml)

Helichrysum	4 drops
Tangerine	4 drops
Neroli	2 drops
Carrier oil	2 teaspoons (10 ml)

Lemon	3 drops
Thyme	2 drops
Vanilla (CO_2)	2 drops
Grapefruit	2 drops
Patchouli	1 drop
Carrier oil	2 teaspoons (10 ml)

Lemon	3 drops
Helichrysum	3 drops
Basil (Sweet)	2 drops
Neroli	2 drops
Carrier oil	2 teaspoons (10 ml)

Grapefruit	2 drops
Vanilla (CO_2)	2 drops
Lemon	2 drops
Helichrysum	2 drops
Spearmint	2 drops
Carrier oil	2 teaspoons (10 ml)

Basil (Sweet)	2 drops
Cardamom	2 drops
Spearmint	2 drops
Vanilla (CO_2)	2 drops
Lemon	2 drops
Carrier oil	2 teaspoons (10 ml)

Lime	3 drops
Tangerine	3 drops
Spearmint	2 drops
Cedarwood (Atlas)	2 drops
Carrier oil	2 teaspoons (10 ml)

Helichrysum	3 drops
Lime	3 drops
Basil (Sweet)	2 drops
Cabreuva	2 drops
Carrier oil	2 teaspoons (10 ml)

Helichrysum	3 drops
Tangerine	3 drops
Neroli	2 drops
Patchouli	2 drops
Carrier oil	2 teaspoons (10 ml)

Grapefruit	4 drops
Peppermint	4 drops
Sandalwood	2 drops
Carrier oil	2 teaspoons (10 ml)

Confidence for a Meeting—Inhaler

Choose one of these formulas. Combine the essential oils in a small glass bottle with a wide opening. Inhale the vapors slowly and deeply. Then tightly cap the bottle after using.

Allspice Berry	15 drops
Tangerine	15 drops
Vanilla (CO_2)	3 drops

Spearmint	20 drops
Cedarwood (Atlas)	5 drops

Helichrysum	13 drops
Spearmint	10 drops
Vanilla (CO_2)	5 drops

Litsea Cubeba	10 drops
Peppermint	10 drops
Vanilla (CO_2)	5 drops

DREAMS

Dreams are the windows to our subconscious mind, providing us with hidden messages and invaluable insights and information for what we need to know, learn, and accomplish. Try these dream formulas and see what is revealed.

Dreams—Application

Apply one of these formulas to the wrists, upper chest, and back of the neck, until the oil has been fully absorbed into the skin. Bring the wrists close to the nose and breathe the vapors in deeply. When done, if you wish, dab on cornstarch to dry off any remaining oil.

Use the formula before going to sleep. If you do not dream the first night, repeat the application the following nights. For some people, it may take several applications before obtaining desired results.

Neroli	3 drops
Mandarin	3 drops
Dill	2 drops
Clary Sage	2 drops
Carrier Oil	2 teaspoons (10 ml)

Lemon	3 drops
Cabreuva	2 drops
Chamomile (Roman)	2 drops
Mandarin	2 drops
Cinnamon Leaf	1 drop
Carrier Oil	2 teaspoons (10 ml)

Tangerine	3 drops
Chamomile (Roman)	3 drops
Frankincense	3 drops
Guaiacwood	1 drop
Carrier Oil	2 teaspoons (10 ml)

Cinnamon Leaf	3 drops
Basil (Sweet)	3 drops
Helichrysum	3 drops
Rosemary	1 drop
Carrier Oil	2 teaspoons (10 ml)

Mandarin	3 drops
Basil (Sweet)	3 drops
Frankincense	2 drops
Vanilla (CO_2)	2 drops
Carrier Oil	2 teaspoons (10 ml)

Mandarin	3 drops
Basil (Sweet)	3 drops
Vanilla (CO_2)	3 drops
Nutmeg	1 drop
Carrier Oil	2 teaspoons (10 ml)

Spruce	3 drops
Fir Needles	3 drops
Cypress	2 drops
Lemon	2 drops
Carrier Oil	2 teaspoons (10 ml)

Tangerine	3 drops
Chamomile (Roman)	2 drops
Spruce	2 drops
Anise	2 drops
Nutmeg	1 drop
Carrier Oil	2 teaspoons (10 ml)

Tangerine	4 drops
Clary Sage	3 drops
Neroli	3 drops
Carrier Oil	2 teaspoons (10 ml)

Tangerine	4 drops
Basil (Sweet)	3 drops
Clary Sage	3 drops
Carrier Oil	2 teaspoons (10 ml)

Frankincense	3 drops
Helichrysum	3 drops
Clary Sage	2 drops
Cinnamon Leaf	2 drops
Carrier Oil	2 teaspoons (10 ml)

Vetiver	3 drops
Lemon	3 drops
Frankincense	3 drops
Rosemary	1 drop
Carrier Oil	2 teaspoons (10 ml)

EXPRESS GRATITUDE

We often go through life not clearly communicating to people how much we appreciate them and the good they do for us. Now we can take this extraordinary opportunity to let the special people around us know exactly how we feel.

- Select one of these methods: application, inhaler, or mist spray; and choose a formula.

- Find a quiet, comfortable place to relax where you will not be disturbed, play soft music (optional), and use the formula. Spend about 20 to 30 minutes thinking of the people to whom you would like to express your gratitude. On a sheet of paper, list their names and what you'd like to tell each person. Then phone, write, or communicate in person your gratitude to each of the people you have chosen. After taking action, write the results, and spend time reflecting on what you learned from this experience.

- Repeat this exercise as often as you feel necessary.

Express Gratitude—Application

Apply one of these formulas to the wrists, upper chest, and back of the neck, until the oil has been fully absorbed into the skin. Bring your wrists close to your nose and breathe the vapors in deeply. When done, if you wish, dab on cornstarch to dry off any remaining oil.

Spruce	4 drops
Chamomile (Roman)	3 drops
Lemon	3 drops
Carrier Oil	2 teaspoons (10 ml)

Geranium	3 drops
Lemon	3 drops
Ylang-Ylang	3 drops
Chamomile (Roman)	1 drop
Carrier Oil	2 teaspoons (10 ml)

Tangerine	4 drops
Guaiacwood	2 drops
Anise	2 drops
Vanilla (CO_2)	2 drops
Carrier Oil	2 teaspoons (10 ml)

Spruce	4 drops
Cinnamon Leaf	3 drops
Vanilla (CO_2)	3 drops
Carrier Oil	2 teaspoons (10 ml)

Express Gratitude—Inhaler

Choose one of these formulas. Combine the essential oils in a small glass bottle with a wide opening. Inhale the vapors slowly and deeply. Then tightly cap the bottle after using.

Spruce	25 drops
Lemon	10 drops

Spruce	20 drops
Vanilla (CO_2)	5 drops

Lemon	20 drops
Ylang-Ylang	10 drops

Tangerine	15 drops
Cinnamon Leaf	10 drops
Vanilla (CO_2)	5 drops

Express Gratitude—Mist Spray

Choose one of these formulas. Fill a fine-mist spray bottle with 2 ounces (60 ml) of purified water, add the essential oils, tighten the cap, and shake well. Mist numerous times over the head with eyes closed. Breathe the vapors in slowly and deeply.

Spruce	20 drops
Chamomile (Roman)	20 drops
Lemon	20 drops
Cedarwood (Atlas)	15 drops
Pure Water	2 ounces (60 ml)

Tangerine	35 drops
Spruce	20 drops
Fir Needles	20 drops
Pure Water	2 ounces (60 ml)

Tangerine	20 drops
Lemon	15 drops
Grapefruit	15 drops
Cedarwood (Atlas)	10 drops
Citronella	10 drops
Cinnamon Leaf	5 drops
Pure Water	2 ounces (60 ml)

Chamomile (Roman)	20 drops
Ylang-Ylang	20 drops
Lemongrass	15 drops
Grapefruit	15 drops
Cinnamon Leaf	5 drops
Pure Water	2 ounces (60 ml)

HEART-TO-HEART TALK

When you are sincere, words can come easier from the heart and have the ability to touch another person's heart. This can open greater communication pathways that have not been reached before, help unite people, and bring them closer with more understanding for one another. The formulas here are specific for female and male. If two females want to do the exercise, like a mother and daughter or two sisters, a female formula can be used on each one. Any two formulas for females can be used.

Heart-to-Heart Talk—Application

Apply one of these formulas to the wrists, upper chest, and back of the neck, until the oil has been fully absorbed into the skin. Bring your wrists close to your nose and breathe the vapors in deeply. When done, if you wish, dab on cornstarch to dry off any remaining oil.

Formulas for Females

Neroli	3 drops
Vanilla (CO_2)	3 drops
Tangerine	2 drops
Rose	2 drops
Carrier Oil	2 teaspoons (10 ml)

Neroli	3 drops
Bergamot	3 drops
Ylang-Ylang	2 drops
Anise	2 drops
Carrier Oil	2 teaspoons (10 ml)

Champaca Flower	3 drops
Vanilla (CO_2)	3 drops
Rose	2 drops
Cedarwood (Atlas)	2 drops
Carrier Oil	2 teaspoons (10 ml)

Rose	3 drops
Neroli	3 drops
Cedarwood (Atlas)	2 drops
Cinnamon Leaf	2 drops
Carrier Oil	2 teaspoons (10 ml)

Vanilla (CO_2)	3 drops
Bergamot	3 drops
Anise	2 drops
Rose	2 drops
Carrier Oil	2 teaspoons (10 ml)

Bergamot	4 drops
Sandalwood	4 drops
Ylang-Ylang	2 drops
Carrier Oil	2 teaspoons (10 ml)

Formulas for Males

Spruce	4 drops
Spearmint	2 drops
Tangerine	2 drops
Sandalwood	2 drops
Carrier Oil	2 teaspoons (10 ml)

Vanilla (CO_2)	4 drops
Spruce	4 drops
Sandalwood	2 drops
Carrier Oil	2 teaspoons (10 ml)

Vanilla (CO_2)	4 drops
Tangerine	2 drops
Fir Needles	2 drops
Spearmint	2 drops
Carrier Oil	2 teaspoons (10 ml)

Litsea Cubeba	2 drops
Mandarin	2 drops
Spruce	2 drops
Galbanum	2 drops
Vanilla (CO_2)	2 drops
Carrier Oil	2 teaspoons (10 ml)

Spruce	4 drops
Sandalwood	3 drops
Vanilla (CO_2)	3 drops
Carrier Oil	2 teaspoons (10 ml)

Fir Needles	3 drops
Spruce	3 drops
Spearmint	2 drops
Vanilla (CO_2)	2 drops
Carrier Oil	2 teaspoons (10 ml)

Heart-To-Heart Talk—Inhaler

Choose one of these formulas. Combine the essential oils in a small glass bottle with a wide opening. Inhale the vapors slowly and deeply. Then tightly cap the bottle after using.

Formulas for Females

Vanilla (CO_2)	10 drops
Rose	3 drops
Tangerine	15 drops
Rose	3 drops

Formulas for Males

Spruce	10 drops
Spearmint	10 drops
Vanilla (CO_2)	5 drops
Fir Needles	10 drops
Litsea Cubeba	10 drops
Spruce	10 drops
Sandalwood	5 drops

Heart-To-Heart Talk—Mist Spray

Choose one of these formulas. Fill a fine-mist spray bottle with 2 ounces (60 ml) of purified water, add the essential oils, tighten the cap, and shake well. Mist numerous times over the head with eyes closed. Breathe the vapors in slowly and deeply.

Formulas for Females

Orange	20 drops
Bergamot	20 drops
Anise	15 drops
Neroli	10 drops
Rose	10 drops
Pure Water	2 ounces (60 ml)
Litsea Cubeba	25 drops
Guaiacwood	20 drops
Rose	10 drops
Neroli	10 drops
Vanilla (CO_2)	10 drops
Pure Water	2 ounces (60 ml)
Tangerine	40 drops
Petitgrain	20 drops
Vanilla (CO_2)	10 drops
Rose	5 drops
Pure Water	2 ounces (60 ml)
Citronella	40 drops
Ylang-Ylang	20 drops
Petitgrain	10 drops
Patchouli	5 drops
Pure Water	2 ounces (60 ml)
Petitgrain	20 drops
Neroli	20 drops
Orange	15 drops
Lemon	15 drops
Rose	5 drops
Pure Water	2 ounces (60 ml)
Litsea Cubeba	30 drops
Orange	20 drops
Vanilla (CO_2)	10 drops
Rose	5 drops
Cinnamon Leaf	5 drops
Vetiver	5 drops
Pure Water	2 ounces (60 ml)

Formulas for Males

Spruce	30 drops
Spearmint	18 drops
Tangerine	17 drops
Sandalwood	10 drops
Pure Water	2 ounces (60 ml)

Spruce	30 drops
Tangerine	20 drops
Fir Needles	15 drops
Vanilla (CO_2)	10 drops
Pure Water	2 ounces (60 ml)

Spearmint	25 drops
Fir Needles	20 drops
Tangerine	15 drops
Amyris	15 drops
Pure Water	2 ounces (60 ml)

Spruce	30 drops
Litsea Cubeba	25 drops
Vanilla (CO_2)	15 drops
Mandarin	5 drops
Pure Water	2 ounces (60 ml)

Fir Needles	25 drops
Tangerine	15 drops
Vanilla (CO_2)	15 drops
Citronella	10 drops
Amyris	10 drops
Pure Water	2 ounces (60 ml)

Spruce	25 drops
Litsea Cubeba	25 drops
Cedarwood (Atlas)	15 drops
Vanilla (CO_2)	10 drops
Pure Water	2 ounces (60 ml)

LAZINESS RELIEF

Most people experience times when they feel sluggish, find it difficult to get going, and don't accomplish the work that needs to be done. Select and use one of these application formulas on yourself or another person to help get out of a lazy state.

Laziness Relief—Application

Apply one of these formulas to the wrists, upper chest, and back of the neck, until the oil has been fully absorbed into the skin. Bring your wrists close to your nose and breathe the vapors in deeply. When done, if you wish, dab on cornstarch to dry off any remaining oil.

Spearmint	4 drops
Hyssop Decumbens	2 drops
Fennel (Sweet)	2 drops
Patchouli	2 drops
Carrier Oil	2 teaspoons (10 ml)

Helichrysum	4 drops
Lemon	2 drops
Thyme	2 drops
Rosemary	2 drops
Carrier Oil	2 teaspoons (10 ml)

Helichrysum	4 drops
Rosemary	3 drops
Vanilla (CO_2)	3 drops
Carrier Oil	2 teaspoons (10 ml)

Sage (Spanish)	3 drops
Lemongrass	3 drops
Peppermint	3 drops
Patchouli	1 drop
Carrier Oil	2 teaspoons (10 ml)

Peppermint	3 drops
Rosemary	3 drops
Patchouli	2 drops
Helichrysum	2 drops
Carrier Oil	2 teaspoons (10 ml)

Peppermint	4 drops
Sage (Spanish)	2 drops
Helichrysum	2 drops
Vanilla (CO_2)	2 drops
Carrier Oil	2 teaspoons (10 ml)

Helichrysum	3 drops
Neroli	3 drops
Vanilla (CO_2)	2 drops
Patchouli	2 drops
Carrier Oil	2 teaspoons (10 ml)

Peppermint	4 drops
Thyme	3 drops
Vanilla (CO_2)	3 drops
Carrier Oil	2 teaspoons (10 ml)

Spearmint	3 drops
Vanilla (CO_2)	3 drops
Fennel (Sweet)	2 drops
Rosemary	2 drops
Carrier Oil	2 teaspoons (10 ml)

Spearmint	3 drops
Helichrysum	3 drops
Cabreuva	2 drops
Ravensara Aromatica	2 drops
Carrier Oil	2 teaspoons (10 ml)

MAKE A DIFFERENCE

All of us would like to see the world we live in become a better place. One good person can truly make a big difference in the lives of others. Think back to when you were younger and how a good person was a positive influence on your life. Think of how important this person was to you and all the good memories you have. Now you can play the same meaningful role with other people in your life who need positive guidance. This could turn out to be the greatest gift you'll ever give.

- Select one of these methods: application, inhaler, or mist spray; and choose a formula.

- Find a quiet, comfortable place to relax where you will not be disturbed, play soft music (optional), and use the formula. Close your eyes and spend about 20 to 30 minutes reflecting back, and thinking of the fond memories you have of a person who was a great influence in your life. Spend some time to capture these wonderful feelings. Afterward, think about the people in your life now who can benefit greatly from your guidance. On a sheet of paper, list the people you can give positive guidance to and how you will accomplish this. After you've made a difference in someone's life, write down the results and how you felt about your achievement.

- Do this exercise frequently to make a difference in someone's life.

Make a Difference—Application

Apply one of these formulas to the wrists, upper chest, and back of the neck, until the oil has been fully absorbed into the skin. Bring your wrists close to your nose and breathe the vapors in deeply. When done, if you wish, dab on cornstarch to dry off any remaining oil.

Peppermint	4 drops
Vanilla (CO_2)	4 drops
Thyme	2 drops
Carrier Oil	2 teaspoons (10 ml)

Helichrysum	5 drops
Spearmint	3 drops
Spikenard	2 drops
Carrier Oil	2 teaspoons (10 ml)

Spruce	4 drops
Vanilla (CO_2)	4 drops
Cedarwood (Atlas)	2 drops
Carrier Oil	2 teaspoons (10 ml)

Orange	4 drops
Lemon	3 drops
Rosewood	3 drops
Carrier Oil	2 teaspoons (10 ml)

Orange	4 drops
Chamomile (Roman)	4 drops
Allspice Berry	2 drops
Carrier Oil	2 teaspoons (10 ml)

Cedarwood (Atlas)	4 drops
Chamomile (Roman)	4 drops
Lime	2 drops
Carrier Oil	2 teaspoons (10 ml)

Make a Difference—Inhaler

Choose one of these formulas. Combine the essential oils in a small glass bottle with a wide opening. Inhale the vapors slowly and deeply. Then tightly cap the bottle after using.

| Lime | 20 drops |
| Vanilla (CO_2) | 5 drops |

Orange	20 drops
Neroli	5 drops
Rose	3 drops

| Spearmint | 25 drops |
| Vanilla (CO_2) | 5 drops |

Helichrysum	20 drops
Spearmint	10 drops
Rose	3 drops

Orange	20 drops
Rosewood	5 drops
Rose	2 drops

| Peppermint | 25 drops |
| Rosewood | 5 drops |

Make a Difference—Mist Spray

Choose one of these formulas. Fill a fine-mist spray bottle with 2 ounces (60 ml) of purified water, add the essential oils, tighten the cap, and shake well. Mist numerous times over the head with eyes closed. Breathe the vapors in slowly and deeply.

Peppermint	20 drops
Orange	20 drops
Clove Bud	15 drops
Lemon	10 drops
Cedarwood (Atlas)	10 drops
Pure Water	2 ounces (60 ml)

Spearmint	30 drops
Thyme	15 drops
Orange	15 drops
Cedarwood (Atlas)	15 drops
Pure Water	2 ounces (60 ml)

Spruce	20 drops
Lemon	20 drops
Grapefruit	15 drops
Clove Bud	15 drops
Spikenard	5 drops
Pure Water	2 ounces (60 ml)

Lemon	20 drops
Eucalyptus Radiata	20 drops
Orange	15 drops
Chamomile (Roman)	10 drops
Spruce	10 drops
Pure Water	2 ounces (60 ml)

MELANCHOLY RELIEF

There are times when things don't go as well as planned and a person may become discouraged. When this happens, take a break from what you are doing and use one of these application formulas.

Melancholy Relief—Application

Relax in a comfortable chair and apply the carrier oil on one palm of the hand. Gently rub the palms together to spread the oil evenly. Then place the essential oils over the carrier oil and rub in well. Close your eyes; cup both hands and raise them close to your nose and breathe in slowly and deeply for about ten minutes. If you need additional drops of carrier oil, apply it. After the completion of the inhalation, dab some cornstarch on one palm and rub both palms together to dry any remaining oil on the skin. Enjoy the experience.

Peppermint	1 drop
Tangerine	1 drop
Carrier Oil	6 drops

Bergamot	1 drop
Ylang-Ylang	1 drop
Carrier Oil	6 drops

Helichrysum	1 drop
Neroli	1 drop
Carrier Oil	6 drops

Champaca Flower	1 drop
Amyris	1 drop
Carrier Oil	6 drops

Rose	1 drop
Sandalwood	1 drop
Carrier Oil	6 drops

Vanilla (CO_2)	1 drop
Frankincense	1 drop
Carrier Oil	6 drops

Ylang-Ylang	1 drop
Amyris	1 drop
Carrier Oil	6 drops

Vanilla (CO_2)	1 drop
Neroli	1 drop
Carrier Oil	6 drops

Spearmint	1 drop
Vanilla (CO_2)	1 drop
Carrier Oil	6 drops

Neroli	1 drop
Tangerine	1 drop
Carrier Oil	6 drops

Vanilla (CO_2)	1 drop
Tangerine	1 drop
Carrier Oil	6 drops

Vanilla (CO_2)	1 drop
Palmarosa	1 drop
Carrier Oil	6 drops

MORNING AFFIRMATION

When arising in the morning, take a few minutes to get the day started right with a positive mind-set. Select and use one of the application or inhaler formulas and reflect on the *Morning Affirmation*.

Morning Affirmation—Application

Choose one of these formulas. Apply the carrier oil on the wrist. Gently rub both wrists together to spread the oil evenly. Then place the essential oils over the carrier oil and rub in well. Bring both wrists close to your nose and breathe the vapors in deeply. If you need additional drops of carrier oil, apply it. Say the *Morning Affirmation*. Afterward, if you wish, dab some cornstarch on one wrist and rub both wrists together to dry any remaining oil on the skin.

Champaca Flower	2 drops
Vanilla (CO_2)	1 drop
Carrier Oil	8 drops
Helichrysum	2 drops
Neroli	1 drop
Carrier Oil	8 drops
Vanilla (CO_2)	2 drops
Sandalwood	1 drop
Carrier Oil	8 drops

Morning Affirmation

Today is special. I give thanks for being granted another precious day of life. I am grateful for having enough food to eat, clothing to wear, a shelter to live in, and people and pets who love me.

I cherish my freedom to do as I wish and go where I want. There are many individuals in this world who are not as fortunate as I am, who lack these vital necessities.

I uphold high standards, values, and principles. The choices and decisions I make are based on reality and truth. I am willing to correct my beliefs or thinking, should I find them to be faulty.

I conduct myself with utmost integrity. I take full responsibility for all my actions. Should I make mistakes, I use them as a learning experience to help me grow wiser, and improve the quality of my life.

Let this precious day not pass without my having acquired new beneficial knowledge and done kind deeds. I realize that every good deed I do for others, not only benefits them, but also helps me feel good about myself.

I set a positive example and serve as a role model for others to follow. By being as good as I can be, I do my share to make this a better world.

From this day forward, I will carry out my responsibilities to the best of my ability, and extend love, kindness, consideration, respect, and understanding to all living beings around me.

I am now ready to do everything I can possibility do to have a great day.

Tangerine	2 drops
Neroli	1 drop
Carrier Oil	8 drops

Tangerine	2 drops
Rose	1 drop
Carrier Oil	8 drops

Champaca Flower	2 drops
Chamomile (Roman)	1 drop
Carrier Oil	8 drops

Morning Affirmation—Inhaler

Choose one of these formulas. Combine the essential oils in a small glass bottle with a wide opening. Inhale the vapors slowly and deeply. Then tightly cap the bottle after using. Say the *Morning Affirmation.*

Spearmint	12 drops
Vanilla (CO_2)	4 drops

Neroli	8 drops
Helichrysum	8 drops

Tangerine	10 drops
Rose	5 drops

Champaca Flowers	8 drops
Chamomile (Roman)	8 drops

OPEN YOUR HEART FOR LOVE

Many of us have been close to relatives or friends and later on the relationships turned out to be very hurtful and caused great pain. As a result of these harmful experiences, we may have closed off an important part of ourselves that enables us to get close to and love another person. If you feel ready now to release those hurtful feelings and let them go, select one of the application formulas and do the exercise.

- Find a quiet, comfortable place to relax where you will not be disturbed, play soft music (optional), and apply the formula. Close your eyes and spend about 20 to 30 minutes thinking about the people and the hurtful feelings you want to let go of. Write down on a sheet of paper, the following: *I am now ready to open my heart for love and relinquish my hurt and painful feelings that were caused by the following people.* Then list the individuals and the hurtful feelings connected with them. Allow those feelings to pass by giving yourself permission to release them. Breathe the oils in deeply and fully exhale out. Slowly deepen the breath. Continue to release and let go.

- For best results, you may need to repeat this exercise several times. Write down the positive changes that have occurred in your life due to letting go of those hurtful feelings.

Open Your Heart for Love— Application

Apply one of these formulas to the wrists, upper chest, and back of the neck, until the oil has been fully absorbed into the skin. Bring your wrists close to your nose and breathe the vapors in deeply. When done, if you wish, dab on cornstarch to dry off any remaining oil.

Sandalwood	3 drops
Orange	3 drops
Vanilla (CO_2)	3 drops
Rose	1 drop
Carrier Oil	2 teaspoons (10 ml)

Spearmint	3 drops
Neroli	3 drops
Orange	3 drops
Cedarwood (Atlas)	1 drop
Carrier Oil	2 teaspoons (10 ml)

Champaca Flower	3 drops
Lime	3 drops
Orange	2 drops
Vanilla (CO_2)	2 drops
Carrier Oil	2 teaspoons (10 ml)

Ylang-Ylang	3 drops
Litsea Cubeba	3 drops
Lemon	2 drops
Clove Bud	2 drops
Carrier Oil	2 teaspoons (10 ml)

PRACTICE KINDNESS

Goodness exists in each and every one of us. But when a person lives in a fast-paced, stressful society such as ours, the pressures of everyday life can often suppress many of our warm, compassionate, kind, and loving feelings.

- Select one of these methods: application, inhaler, or mist spray; and choose a formula.

- Find a quiet, comfortable place to relax where you will not be disturbed, play soft music (optional), and use the formula. Spend about 20 to 30 minutes thinking about kind deeds to do in order to derive inner satisfaction without expecting anything in return. For example, feed a hungry animal, plant a berry bush to provide food for the birds, go out of your way for a deserving person, or do something special for someone you care about.

The acts of kindness should involve giving of yourself and not any material gifts. On a sheet of paper, list the acts of kindness you plan to do. After completing each one, write down how it made you feel and the results of your action. When you accomplish all the *Practice Kindness* deeds on the list, reflect on what you've learned from this exercise, and write that as your conclusion.

- Repeat this exercise often.

Practice Kindness—Application

Apply one of these formulas to the wrists, upper chest, and back of the neck, until the oil has been fully absorbed into the skin. Bring your wrists close to your nose and breathe the vapors in deeply. When done, if you wish, dab on cornstarch to dry off any remaining oil.

Tangerine	4 drops
Cedarwood (Atlas)	3 drops
Helichrysum	3 drops
Carrier Oil	2 teaspoons (10 ml)

Orange	4 drops
Neroli	3 drops
Helichrysum	3 drops
Carrier Oil	2 teaspoons (10 ml)

Rosewood	4 drops
Neroli	3 drops
Vanilla (CO_2)	3 drops
Carrier Oil	2 teaspoons (10 ml)

Tangerine	4 drops
Lemongrass	4 drops
Patchouli	2 drops
Carrier Oil	2 teaspoons (10 ml)

Spruce	4 drops
Tangerine	4 drops
Frankincense	2 drops
Carrier Oil	2 teaspoons (10 ml)

Clary Sage	3 drops
Vanilla (CO_2)	3 drops
Spearmint	2 drops
Copaiba	2 drops
Carrier Oil	2 teaspoons (10 ml)

Geranium	4 drops
Allspice Berry	3 drops
Lemon	3 drops
Carrier Oil	2 teaspoons (10 ml)

Helichrysum	4 drops
Cardamom	3 drops
Neroli	3 drops
Carrier Oil	2 teaspoons (10 ml)

Helichrysum	4 drops
Palmarosa	4 drops
Allspice Berry	2 drops
Carrier Oil	2 teaspoons (10 ml)

Geranium	4 drops
Grapefruit	2 drops
Orange	2 drops
Allspice Berry	2 drops
Carrier Oil	2 teaspoons (10 ml)

Helichrysum	4 drops
Ylang-Ylang	2 drops
Palmarosa	2 drops
Lemon	2 drops
Carrier Oil	2 teaspoons (10 ml)

Geranium	3 drops
Ylang-Ylang	3 drops
Allspice Berry	2 drops
Spikenard	2 drops
Carrier Oil	2 teaspoons (10 ml)

Practice Kindness—Inhaler

Choose one of these formulas. Combine the essential oils in a small glass bottle with a wide opening. Inhale the vapors slowly and deeply. Then tightly cap the bottle after using.

Ylang-Ylang	10 drops
Citronella	10 drops

Champaca Flower	10 drops
Vetiver	3 drops
Vanilla (CO_2)	3 drops

Mandarin	10 drops
Grapefruit	10 drops
Rose	3 drops

Grapefruit	20 drops
Neroli	7 drops
Dill	5 drops

Litsea Cubeba	10 drops
Vanilla (CO_2)	5 drops

Ylang-Ylang	8 drops
Palmarosa	5 drops
Citronella	5 drops
Clove Bud	5 drops

Practice Kindness—Mist Spray

Choose one of these formulas. Fill a fine-mist spray bottle with 2 ounces (60 ml) of purified water, add the essential oils, tighten the cap, and shake well. Mist numerous times over the head with eyes closed. Breathe the vapors in slowly and deeply.

Litsea Cubeba	25 drops
Orange	25 drops
Lime	20 drops
Cinnamon Leaf	5 drops
Pure Water	2 ounces (60 ml)

Petitgrain	20 drops
Orange	18 drops
Tangerine	17 drops
Lemongrass	10 drops
Amyris	10 drops
Pure Water	2 ounces (60 ml)

Rosewood	25 drops
Tangerine	25 drops
Lemongrass	20 drops
Patchouli	5 drops
Pure Water	2 ounces (60 ml)

Grapefruit	20 drops
Ylang-Ylang	20 drops
Litsea Cubeba	20 drops
Lemon	10 drops
Cedarwood (Atlas)	5 drops
Pure Water	2 ounces (60 ml)

Palmarosa	18 drops
Orange	18 drops
Grapefruit	18 drops
Lemon	11 drops
Cardamom	10 drops
Pure Water	2 ounces (60 ml)

Geranium	20 drops
Ylang-Ylang	15 drops
Clove Bud	15 drops
Lemon	15 drops
Grapefruit	10 drops
Pure Water	2 ounces (60 ml)

RECOGNIZE YOUR TREASURES

A true state of happiness can only be attained when a person is grateful and appreciative. We shouldn't have to starve in order to appreciate the food we have to eat, become homeless to appreciate our home, or wait until we lose a loved one to realize how precious the person was to us.

Count your blessings. Be grateful for what you have!

• Select one of these methods: application or mist spray; and choose a formula.

• Find a quiet, comfortable room to relax where you will not be disturbed, play soft music (optional), and use the formula. Close your eyes and spend about 20 to 30 minutes thinking about everything in your life that you should treasure and all that you have to be thankful for. On a sheet of paper, list the treasures you need to be grateful for and appreciative of. Then write a plan of action to make important changes to recognize the treasures in your life. For example, the action plan for appreciating having enough food to eat would be not to waste food. To treasure the beauty of nature and animals, the action plan would be to use natural products that are in harmony with the earth to eliminate harm done to the environment.

• Repeat this exercise often.

Recognize Your Treasures—Application

Apply one of these formulas to the wrists, upper chest, and back of the neck, until the oil has been fully absorbed into the skin. Bring your wrists close to your nose and breathe the vapors in deeply. When done, if you wish, dab on cornstarch to dry off any remaining oil.

Ylang-Ylang	3 drops
Allspice Berry	3 drops
Cedarwood (Atlas)	2 drops
Lemon	2 drops
Carrier Oil	2 teaspoons (10 ml)

Helichrysum	4 drops
Spearmint	3 drops
Orange	3 drops
Carrier Oil	2 teaspoons (10 ml)

Tangerine	4 drops
Vanilla (CO_2)	3 drops
Allspice Berry	3 drops
Carrier Oil	2 teaspoons (10 ml)

Chamomile (Roman)	3 drops
Helichrysum	3 drops
Cedarwood (Atlas)	2 drops
Spearmint	2 drops
Carrier Oil	2 teaspoons (10 ml)

Recognize Your Treasures—Mist Spray

Choose one of these formulas. Fill a fine-mist spray bottle with 2 ounces (60 ml) of purified water, add the essential oils, tighten the cap, and shake well. Mist numerous times over the head with eyes closed. Breathe the vapors in slowly and deeply.

Tangerine	40 drops
Clove Bud	20 drops
Lemongrass	15 drops
Pure Water	2 ounces (60 ml)

Orange	40 drops
Helichrysum	20 drops
Lemon	8 drops
Cedarwood (Atlas)	7 drops
Pure Water	2 ounces (60 ml)

Spearmint	35 drops
Spruce	20 drops
Eucalyptus Radiata	10 drops
Citronella	10 drops
Pure Water	2 ounces (60 ml)

Orange	40 drops
Grapefruit	15 drops
Rosewood	10 drops
Cinnamon Leaf	5 drops
Citronella	5 drops
Pure Water	2 ounces (60 ml)

WAKE UP TO A GREAT DAY!

It is so important to wake up feeling refreshed, rejuvenated, and in a positive state, ready to have a great day. Select and use one of the diffuser or mist spray formulas, and get your day started right!

Wake Up to a Great Day!—Diffuser

Before going to bed, choose one of these formulas. Depending on the type of diffuser you have, place the essential oils in the designated area of the diffuser. Set an electric timer to turn on the diffuser ten minutes before your alarm clock rings. Connect the diffuser to the timer, and in the morning the reviving aroma will disperse into the air.

Spearmint	100%

Spearmint	60%
Spruce	20%
Tangerine	20%

Spearmint	70%
Spruce	20%
Thyme	10%

Peppermint	80%
Rosemary	20%

Peppermint	80%
Lime	20%

Grapefruit	25%
Lemon	25%
Orange	25%
Tangerine	25%

Wake Up to a Great Day!—Mist Spray

Choose one of these formulas. Fill a fine-mist spray bottle with 2 ounces (60 ml) of purified water, add the essential oils, tighten the cap,

and shake well. Mist numerous times over the head with eyes closed. Breathe the vapors in slowly and deeply.

Spearmint	55 drops
Cedarwood (Atlas)	20 drops
Pure Water	2 ounces (60 ml)

Spearmint	50 drops
Eucalyptus Radiata	15 drops
Lemon	10 drops
Pure Water	2 ounces (60 ml)

Spearmint	45 drops
Spruce	20 drops
Thyme	10 drops
Pure Water	2 ounces (60 ml)

Grapefruit	25 drops
Lemon	20 drops
Orange	20 drops
Cedarwood (Atlas)	10 drops
Pure Water	2 ounces (60 ml)

CHAPTER 6

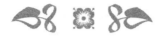

Massage

Massage is the oldest and one of the most effective forms of therapy. Its healing power was well known in ancient times. Hippocrates, the father of medicine, in fourth-century B.C. Greece, advocated that people receive a massage to maintain good health.

Enjoying touch is one way to experience a state of worthiness and well-being. Touching is one of the simplest ways to convey and receive feelings of compassion, warmth, closeness, and love.

When the essential oils are combined with the therapeutic value of a massage, the experience is greatly enhanced. Exchanging aromatherapy massages with friends and loved ones can help us not only feel great but also satisfy our vital need for touch.

BACK RENEW

Massage one of these formulas into the back for at least 30 minutes and until the oil is fully absorbed into the skin. After the massage, dab on cornstarch to dry off any remaining oil.

Helichrysum	5 drops
Cabreuva	3 drops
Thyme	3 drops
Cedarwood (Atlas)	2 drops
Tangerine	2 drops
Carrier Oil	1 tablespoon (15 ml)

Rosewood	4 drops
Helichrysum	4 drops
Lime	4 drops
Tangerine	2 drops
Allspice Berry	1 drop
Carrier Oil	1 tablespoon (15 ml)

Geranium	4 drops
Helichrysum	4 drops
Thyme	3 drops
Ginger	2 drops
Rosemary	2 drops
Carrier Oil	1 tablespoon (15 ml)

Geranium	4 drops
Cabreuva	3 drops
Guaiacwood	3 drops
Allspice Berry	3 drops
Lemon	2 drops
Carrier Oil	1 tablespoon (15 ml)

Ylang-Ylang	4 drops
Allspice Berry	3 drops
Amyris	3 drops
Marjoram	3 drops
Helichrysum	2 drops
Carrier Oil	1 tablespoon (15 ml)

Ylang-Ylang	4 drops
Spikenard	4 drops
Spearmint	3 drops
Palmarosa	2 drops
Cumin	2 drops
Carrier Oil	1 tablespoon (15 ml)

Helichrysum	4 drops
Ylang-Ylang	4 drops
Spikenard	4 drops
Cinnamon Leaf	3 drops
Carrier Oil	1 tablespoon (15 ml)

Amyris	5 drops
Spearmint	5 drops
Thyme	3 drops
Rosemary	2 drops
Carrier Oil	1 tablespoon (15 ml)

BE YOUR OWN BEST FRIEND

When there is no one else around to give you a massage, treat yourself to a self-nurturing application. Massage one of these formulas into the upper chest, back of the neck, and shoulders for at least 30 minutes and until the oil is fully absorbed into the skin. Breathe the vapors in deeply. After the massage, dab on cornstarch to dry off any remaining oil.

Neroli	4 drops
Vanilla (CO_2)	4 drops
Petitgrain	4 drops
Mandarin	3 drops
Carrier Oil	1 tablespoon (15 ml)

Helichrysum	4 drops
Sandalwood	3 drops
Tangerine	3 drops
Lemon	3 drops
Geranium	2 drops
Carrier Oil	1 tablespoon (15 ml)

Champaca Flower	4 drops
Allspice Berry	3 drops
Sandalwood	3 drops
Mandarin	3 drops
Petitgrain	2 drops
Carrier Oil	1 tablespoon (15 ml)

Sandalwood	4 drops
Spearmint	3 drops
Mandarin	3 drops
Allspice Berry	3 drops
Lemon	2 drops
Carrier Oil	1 tablespoon (15 ml)

Helichrysum	4 drops
Eucalyptus Citriodora	4 drops
Vanilla (CO_2)	4 drops
Mandarin	3 drops
Carrier Oil	1 tablespoon (15 ml)

Neroli	4 drops
Mandarin	4 drops
Eucalyptus Citriodora	4 drops
Amyris	3 drops
Carrier Oil	1 tablespoon (15 ml)

Rosewood	4 drops
Mandarin	4 drops
Allspice Berry	4 drops
Lemon	3 drops
Carrier Oil	1 tablespoon (15 ml)

Helichrysum	5 drops
Spearmint	4 drops
Rosewood	3 drops
Eucalyptus Citriodora	3 drops
Carrier Oil	1 tablespoon (15 ml)

Neroli	4 drops
Dill	4 drops
Mandarin	4 drops
Champaca Flower	3 drops
Carrier Oil	1 tablespoon (15 ml)

Helichrysum	5 drops
Neroli	4 drops
Dill	3 drops
Tangerine	3 drops
Carrier Oil	1 tablespoon (15 ml)

GET CLOSER TO SOMEONE YOU LOVE

With our fast-paced lifestyle and the daily struggle of trying to beat the clock to get everything done, we often neglect to spend quality time with the people we care for. To open up a deeper relationship of caring, understanding, and communication, make it a priority to set aside time and give a massage to a loved one: son, daughter, brother, sister, spouse, friend, or anyone you'd like to get closer to. Enjoy the special time together.

Massage one of these formulas into the back of the neck, shoulders, and back for at least 30 minutes and until the oil is fully absorbed into the skin. After the massage, dab on cornstarch to dry off any remaining oil.

Helichrysum	4 drops
Neroli	4 drops
Lime	4 drops
Sandalwood	3 drops
Carrier Oil	1 tablespoon (15 ml)

Tangerine	4 drops
Lime	4 drops
Sandalwood	3 drops
Cinnamon Leaf	2 drops
Rose	2 drops
Carrier Oil	1 tablespoon (15 ml)

Vanilla (CO_2)	4 drops
Allspice Berry	4 drops
Mandarin	4 drops
Lime	3 drops
Carrier Oil	1 tablespoon (15 ml)

Allspice Berry	4 drops
Tangerine	4 drops
Lime	4 drops
Petitgrain	2 drops
Rose	1 drop
Carrier Oil	1 tablespoon (15 ml)

Mandarin	4 drops
Neroli	4 drops
Rosewood	4 drops
Allspice Berry	3 drops
Carrier Oil	1 tablespoon (15 ml)

Lime	5 drops
Mandarin	4 drops
Vanilla (CO_2)	3 drops
Rosewood	3 drops
Carrier Oil	1 tablespoon (15 ml)

Tangerine	4 drops
Sandalwood	4 drops
Lime	4 drops
Spearmint	3 drops
Carrier Oil	1 tablespoon (15 ml)

Mandarin	4 drops
Allspice Berry	4 drops
Neroli	4 drops
Rose	3 drops
Carrier Oil	1 tablespoon (15 ml)

Lemon	5 drops
Allspice Berry	4 drops
Ylang-Ylang	4 drops
Amyris	2 drops
Carrier Oil	1 tablespoon (15 ml)

Lemon	4 drops
Grapefruit	4 drops
Neroli	4 drops
Spearmint	3 drops
Carrier Oil	1 tablespoon (15 ml)

GET UP & GO!

Massage one of these formulas into the upper chest and back of the neck for at least 30 minutes and until the oil is fully absorbed into the skin. After the massage, dab on cornstarch to dry off any remaining oil.

Rosemary	4 drops
Helichrysum	4 drops
Spearmint	4 drops
Vanilla (CO_2)	3 drops
Carrier Oil	1 tablespoon (15 ml)

Peppermint	5 drops
Rosemary	4 drops
Litsea Cubeba	4 drops
Patchouli	2 drops
Carrier Oil	1 tablespoon (15 ml)

Lemongrass	5 drops
Spearmint	5 drops
Helichrysum	5 drops
Carrier Oil	1 tablespoon (15 ml)

Lemongrass	4 drops
Helichrysum	4 drops
Patchouli	4 drops
Fennel (Sweet)	3 drops
Carrier Oil	1 tablespoon (15 ml)

INNER PEACE

If we want to have a peaceful world, we must start with our own inner peace first. Massage one of these formulas into the back of the neck, shoulders, and back for at least 30 minutes and until the oil is fully absorbed into the skin. After the massage, dab on cornstarch to dry off any remaining oil.

Lavender	4 drops
Chamomile (Roman)	3 drops
Mandarin	3 drops
Neroli	3 drops
Amyris	2 drops
Carrier Oil	1 tablespoon (15 ml)

Chamomile (Roman)	4 drops
Ylang-Ylang	3 drops
Vetiver	3 drops
Lemon	3 drops
Champaca Flower	2 drops
Carrier Oil	1 tablespoon (15 ml)

Chamomile (Roman)	4 drops
Marjoram	3 drops
Spikenard	3 drops
Palmarosa	3 drops
Rose	2 drops
Carrier Oil	1 tablespoon (15 ml)

Lavender	3 drops
Mandarin	3 drops
Vanilla (CO_2)	3 drops
Amyris	3 drops
Dill	3 drops
Carrier Oil	1 tablespoon (15 ml)

Chamomile (Roman)	4 drops
Celery	3 drops
Vanilla (CO_2)	3 drops
Mandarin	3 drops
Anise	2 drops
Carrier Oil	1 tablespoon (15 ml)

Lavender	3 drops
Clary Sage	3 drops
Petitgrain	3 drops
Mandarin	3 drops
Sandalwood	3 drops
Carrier Oil	1 tablespoon (15 ml)

Neroli	3 drops
Petitgrain	3 drops
Clary Sage	3 drops
Lavender	3 drops
Lemon	3 drops
Carrier Oil	1 tablespoon (15 ml)

Palmarosa	3 drops
Mandarin	3 drops
Chamomile (Roman)	3 drops
Clary Sage	3 drops
Rosewood	3 drops
Carrier Oil	1 tablespoon (15 ml)

LOOK ON THE BRIGHT SIDE

Sometimes the world we live in can get us down, and we need to pick ourselves up. These formulas can help. Massage one of these formulas into the upper chest, back of the neck, shoulders, and back for at least 30 minutes and until the oil is fully absorbed into the skin. After the massage, dab on cornstarch to dry off any remaining oil.

Spruce	4 drops
Mandarin	4 drops
Vanilla (CO_2)	3 drops
Lemon Myrtle	2 drops
Vetiver	2 drops
Carrier Oil	1 tablespoon (15 ml)

Mandarin	4 drops
Palmarosa	3 drops
Litsea Cubeba	3 drops
Sage (Spanish)	3 drops
Guaiacwood	2 drops
Carrier Oil	1 tablespoon (15 ml)

Lavender	4 drops
Spruce	4 drops
Neroli	4 drops
Rosewood	3 drops
Carrier Oil	1 tablespoon (15 ml)

Mandarin	4 drops
Lemon	4 drops
Palmarosa	3 drops
Clary Sage	2 drops
Rose	2 drops
Carrier Oil	1 tablespoon (15 ml)

Spruce	4 drops
Lavender	4 drops
Frankincense	4 drops
Vanilla (CO$_2$)	3 drops
Carrier Oil	1 tablespoon (15 ml)

Spearmint	3 drops
Helichrysum	3 drops
Mandarin	3 drops
Rosewood	3 drops
Lavender	3 drops
Carrier Oil	1 tablespoon (15 ml)

Palmarosa	4 drops
Frankincense	4 drops
Ylang-Ylang	4 drops
Sage (Spanish)	3 drops
Carrier Oil	1 tablespoon (15 ml)

Mandarin	4 drops
Helichrysum	4 drops
Rose	3 drops
Clary Sage	2 drops
Guaiacwood	2 drops
Carrier Oil	1 tablespoon (15 ml)

Lavender	4 drops
Rose	3 drops
Spearmint	2 drops
Spruce	2 drops
Clary Sage	2 drops
Frankincense	2 drops
Carrier Oil	1 tablespoon (15 ml)

Mandarin	5 drops
Lavender	4 drops
Marjoram	3 drops
Rose	3 drops
Carrier Oil	1 tablespoon (15 ml)

MUSCLE & JOINT EASE

Massage one of these formulas into the muscles and joints, as well as the surrounding areas for at least 30 minutes and until the oil is fully absorbed into the skin. After the massage, dab on cornstarch to dry off any remaining oil. The leftover oil from the formula can be stored for future use. Be sure to label the bottle.

Please note: Another carrier oil can be substituted for evening primrose and/or avocado oil.

Lemon	5 drops
Guaiacwood	4 drops
Thyme	4 drops
Cinnamon Leaf	4 drops
Helichrysum	3 drops
Evening Primrose Oil	2 teaspoons (10 ml)
Avocado Oil	2 teaspoons (10 ml)

Guaiacwood	4 drops
Lime	4 drops
Cajeput	4 drops
Cedarwood (Atlas)	4 drops
Cumin	4 drops
Evening Primrose Oil	2 teaspoons (10 ml)
Avocado Oil	2 teaspoons (10 ml)

Helichrysum	5 drops
Thyme	3 drops
Cumin	3 drops
Lemongrass	3 drops
Galbanum	3 drops
Allspice Berry	3 drops
Evening Primrose Oil	2 teaspoons (10 ml)
Avocado Oil	2 teaspoons (10 ml)

Lemon	5 drops
Helichrysum	5 drops
Rosewood	4 drops
Ginger	3 drops
Marjoram	3 drops
Evening Primrose Oil	2 teaspoons (10 ml)
Avocado Oil	2 teaspoons (10 ml)

Marjoram	5 drops
Helichrysum	5 drops
Ravensara Aromatica	3 drops
Lime	3 drops
Juniper Berry	2 drops
Nutmeg	2 drops
Evening Primrose Oil	2 teaspoons (10 ml)
Avocado Oil	2 teaspoons (10 ml)

Ravensara Aromatica	4 drops
Cabreuva	4 drops
Palmarosa	4 drops
Helichrysum	3 drops
Cinnamon Leaf	3 drops
Lemongrass	2 drops
Evening Primrose Oil	2 teaspoons (10 ml)
Avocado Oil	2 teaspoons (10 ml)

Galbanum	5 drops
Frankincense	4 drops
Lemongrass	4 drops
Thyme	4 drops
Cinnamon Leaf	3 drops
Evening Primrose Oil	2 teaspoons (10 ml)
Avocado Oil	2 teaspoons (10 ml)

Rosewood	4 drops
Thyme	4 drops
Allspice Berry	3 drops
Cabreuva	3 drops
Galbanum	2 drops
Cinnamon Leaf	2 drops
Helichrysum	2 drops
Evening Primrose Oil	2 teaspoons (10 ml)
Avocado Oil	2 teaspoons (10 ml)

PENETRATING CHEST RUB

Massage one of these formulas into the upper chest and back of the neck for at least 30 minutes and until the oil is fully absorbed into the skin. After the massage, dab on cornstarch to dry off any remaining oil.

Thyme	4 drops
Peppermint	3 drops
Black Pepper	3 drops
Carrier Oil	2 teaspoons (10 ml)

Helichrysum	4 drops
Marjoram	4 drops
Black Pepper	2 drops
Carrier Oil	2 teaspoons (10 ml)

Helichrysum	5 drops
Thyme	3 drops
Eucalyptus Radiata	2 drops
Carrier Oil	2 teaspoons (10 ml)

Eucalyptus Radiata	4 drops
Peppermint	3 drops
Ravensara Aromatica	3 drops
Carrier Oil	2 teaspoons (10 ml)

Marjoram	3 drops
Rosemary	3 drops
Spearmint	2 drops
Ginger	2 drops
Carrier Oil	2 teaspoons (10 ml)

Cabreuva	3 drops
Lavender	3 drops
Lemon	2 drops
Cumin	2 drops
Carrier Oil	2 teaspoons (10 ml)

Allspice Berry	3 drops
Lemon	3 drops
Copaiba	2 drops
Peppermint	2 drops
Carrier Oil	2 teaspoons (10 ml)

Myrtle	4 drops
Lavender	3 drops
Marjoram	3 drops
Carrier Oil	2 teaspoons (10 ml)

Allspice Berry	4 drops
Marjoram	4 drops
Thyme	2 drops
Carrier Oil	2 teaspoons (10 ml)

Cabreuva	4 drops
Helichrysum	3 drops
Allspice Berry	3 drops
Carrier Oil	2 teaspoons (10 ml)

QUIET PLEASE!

Some people have a difficult time relaxing while getting a massage. These formulas should help relax and quiet a person so he or she can enjoy the massage.

Massage one of these formulas into the back, back of the neck, and shoulders for at least 30 minutes and until the oil is fully absorbed into the skin. After the massage, dab on cornstarch to dry off any remaining oil.

Dill	4 drops
Neroli	4 drops
Petitgrain	4 drops
Amyris	3 drops
Carrier Oil	1 tablespoon (15 ml)

Dill	3 drops
Marjoram	3 drops
Amyris	3 drops
Celery	3 drops
Orange	3 drops
Carrier Oil	1 tablespoon (15 ml)

Celery	4 drops
Vetiver	4 drops
Petitgrain	4 drops
Marjoram	3 drops
Carrier Oil	1 tablespoon (15 ml)

Copaiba	4 drops
Spikenard	4 drops
Neroli	4 drops
Mandarin	3 drops
Carrier Oil	1 tablespoon (15 ml)

REWARD YOURSELF

These formulas can encourage an overall good feeling for a person who really deserves it. Massage one of these formulas into the back of the neck, shoulders, and entire back for at least 30 minutes and until the oil is fully absorbed into the skin. After the massage, dab on cornstarch to dry off any remaining oil.

Helichrysum	4 drops
Galbanum	4 drops
Mandarin	4 drops
Vanilla (CO_2)	3 drops
Carrier Oil	1 tablespoon (15 ml)

Champaca Flower	4 drops
Litsea Cubeba	3 drops
Ylang-Ylang	3 drops
Palmarosa	3 drops
Patchouli	1 drop
Clove Bud	1 drop
Carrier Oil	1 tablespoon (15 ml)

Neroli	4 drops
Helichrysum	4 drops
Mandarin	4 drops
Champaca Flower	3 drops
Carrier Oil	1 tablespoon (15 ml)

Mandarin	4 drops
Clove Bud	2 drops
Geranium	2 drops
Vanilla (CO_2)	2 drops
Rosewood	2 drops
Amyris	2 drops
Dill	1 drop
Carrier Oil	1 tablespoon (15 ml)

Guaiacwood	4 drops
Ylang-Ylang	3 drops
Grapefruit	3 drops
Galbanum	3 drops
Lemon Myrtle	2 drops
Carrier Oil	1 tablespoon (15 ml)

Helichrysum	3 drops
Mandarin	3 drops
Litsea Cubeba	3 drops
Clove Bud	2 drops
Vetiver	2 drops
Vanilla (CO_2)	2 drops
Carrier Oil	1 tablespoon (15 ml)

Neroli	4 drops
Dill	4 drops
Amyris	3 drops
Champaca Flower	2 drops
Lemon Myrtle	2 drops
Carrier Oil	1 tablespoon (15 ml)

Mandarin	4 drops
Helichrysum	4 drops
Champaca Flower	3 drops
Chamomile (Roman)	2 drops
Guaiacwood	2 drops
Carrier Oil	1 tablespoon (15 ml)

SEVENTH HEAVEN

Use these blends to elevate the mood and promote a state of greater well-being. Massage one of these formulas into the back, back of the neck, upper chest, shoulders, and abdomen for at least 30 minutes and until the oil is fully absorbed into the skin. After the massage, dab on cornstarch to dry off any remaining oil.

Champaca Flower	3 drops
Dill	3 drops
Neroli	3 drops
Clary Sage	3 drops
Vanilla (CO_2)	3 drops
Carrier Oil	1 tablespoon (15 ml)

Geranium	3 drops
Vanilla (CO_2)	3 drops
Tangerine	3 drops
Sandalwood	3 drops
Spearmint	3 drops
Carrier Oil	1 tablespoon (15 ml)

Neroli	4 drops
Dill	3 drops
Lemongrass	3 drops
Helichrysum	3 drops
Cinnamon Leaf	2 drops
Carrier Oil	1 tablespoon (15 ml)

Mandarin	4 drops
Geranium	3 drops
Rosewood	3 drops
Vanilla (CO_2)	3 drops
Litsea Cubeba	2 drops
Carrier Oil	1 tablespoon (15 ml)

SHOULDER & NECK RELEASE

Massage one of these formulas into the upper chest, shoulders, and back of the neck for at least 30 minutes and until the oil is fully absorbed into the skin. After the massage, dab on cornstarch to dry off any remaining oil.

Helichrysum	5 drops
Thyme	4 drops
Galbanum	3 drops
Amyris	3 drops
Carrier Oil	1 tablespoon (15 ml)

Litsea Cubeba	4 drops
Galbanum	4 drops
Amyris	4 drops
Marjoram	3 drops
Carrier Oil	1 tablespoon (15 ml)

Cabreuva	5 drops
Helichrysum	4 drops
Amyris	4 drops
Neroli	2 drops
Carrier Oil	1 tablespoon (15 ml)

Allspice Berry	4 drops
Marjoram	4 drops
Vetiver	4 drops
Galbanum	3 drops
Carrier Oil	1 tablespoon (15 ml)

Amyris	4 drops
Mandarin	4 drops
Thyme	4 drops
Litsea Cubeba	3 drops
Carrier Oil	1 tablespoon (15 ml)

Spruce	4 drops
Fir Needles	4 drops
Marjoram	4 drops
Allspice Berry	3 drops
Carrier Oil	1 tablespoon (15 ml)

Allspice Berry	4 drops
Marjoram	4 drops
Lemon	3 drops
Fennel (Sweet)	3 drops
Vetiver	1 drop
Carrier Oil	1 tablespoon (15 ml)

Allspice Berry	4 drops
Eucalyptus Citriodora	4 drops
Amyris	3 drops
Galbanum	2 drops
Vanilla (CO_2)	2 drops
Carrier Oil	1 tablespoon (15 ml)

Lemon	4 drops
Allspice Berry	3 drops
Ylang-Ylang	3 drops
Palmarosa	3 drops
Galbanum	2 drops
Carrier Oil	1 tablespoon (15 ml)

Amyris	4 drops
Eucalyptus Citriodora	3 drops
Thyme	3 drops
Helichrysum	3 drops
Vanilla (CO_2)	2 drops
Carrier Oil	1 tablespoon (15 ml)

SOOTHE EMOTIONAL UPSET

When having an emotional upset or dealing with an upsetting situation, these formulas can help. Massage one of these formulas into the abdominal area, back of the neck, shoulders, back, and upper chest for at least 30 minutes and until the oil is fully absorbed into the skin. After the massage, dab on cornstarch to dry off any remaining oil.

Chamomile (Roman)	4 drops
Spruce	3 drops
Mandarin	3 drops
Galbanum	3 drops
Rose	2 drops
Carrier Oil	1 tablespoon (15 ml)

Clary Sage	3 drops
Chamomile (Roman)	3 drops
Lavender	3 drops
Vanilla (CO_2)	3 drops
Lemon	3 drops
Carrier Oil	1 tablespoon (15 ml)

Mandarin	4 drops
Chamomile (Roman)	3 drops
Litsea Cubeba	3 drops
Rosewood	3 drops
Vetiver	2 drops
Carrier Oil	1 tablespoon (15 ml)

Chamomile (Roman)	4 drops
Neroli	4 drops
Vanilla (CO_2)	4 drops
Clary Sage	3 drops
Carrier Oil	1 tablespoon (15 ml)

Mandarin	3 drops
Palmarosa	3 drops
Lemon	3 drops
Vetiver	3 drops
Chamomile (Roman)	3 drops
Carrier Oil	1 tablespoon (15 ml)

Neroli	3 drops
Litsea Cubeba	3 drops
Chamomile (Roman)	3 drops
Vanilla (CO_2)	2 drops
Vetiver	2 drops
Dill	2 drops
Carrier Oil	1 tablespoons (15 ml)

SOOTHE HEARTBREAK

When a person experiences heartbreak, it can be a big setback. These formulas can help when used often during this stressful occurrence. Massage one of these formulas into the abdominal area, back of the neck, shoulders, back, and upper chest for at least 30 minutes and until the oil is fully absorbed into the skin. After the massage, dab on cornstarch to dry off any remaining oil.

Lavender	4 drops
Clary Sage	3 drops
Lemon Myrtle	2 drops
Vanilla (CO_2)	2 drops
Amyris	2 drops
Marjoram	2 drops
Carrier Oil	1 tablespoon (15 ml)

Lavender	4 drops
Ylang-Ylang	4 drops
Lemon	3 drops
Amyris	3 drops
Guaiacwood	1 drop
Carrier Oil	1 tablespoon (15 ml)

Clary Sage	3 drops
Tangerine	3 drops
Rose	3 drops
Lavender	3 drops
Litsea Cubeba	3 drops
Carrier Oil	1 tablespoon (15 ml)

Sage (Spanish)	3 drops
Ylang-Ylang	3 drops
Litsea Cubeba	3 drops
Neroli	3 drops
Allspice Berry	3 drops
Carrier Oil	1 tablespoon (15 ml)

Clary Sage	3 drops
Palmarosa	3 drops
Lavender	3 drops
Litsea Cubeba	2 drops
Rose	2 drops
Spikenard	2 drops
Carrier Oil	1 tablespoon (15 ml)

Lemon	4 drops
Ylang-Ylang	3 drops
Helichrysum	3 drops
Galbanum	3 drops
Spikenard	2 drops
Carrier Oil	1 tablespoon (15 ml)

Mandarin	4 drops
Lavender	3 drops
Clary Sage	3 drops
Rose	3 drops
Chamomile (Roman)	2 drops
Carrier Oil	1 tablespoon (15 ml)

Helichrysum	4 drops
Ylang-Ylang	4 drops
Lavender	4 drops
Litsea Cubeba	3 drops
Carrier Oil	1 tablespoon (15 ml)

Marjoram	4 drops
Vetiver	4 drops
Vanilla (CO_2)	4 drops
Mandarin	3 drops
Carrier Oil	1 tablespoon (15 ml)

Sage (Spanish)	3 drops
Vetiver	3 drops
Rose	3 drops
Mandarin	3 drops
Marjoram	3 drops
Carrier Oil	1 tablespoon (15 ml)

SOOTHE NERVOUS TENSION

Massage one of these formulas into the abdominal area, back of the neck, shoulders, back, and upper chest for at least 30 minutes and until the oil is fully absorbed into the skin. After the massage, dab on cornstarch to dry off any remaining oil.

Spikenard	5 drops
Galbanum	4 drops
Neroli	4 drops
Mandarin	2 drops
Carrier Oil	1 tablespoon (15 ml)

Mandarin	4 drops
Petitgrain	4 drops
Lemon	4 drops
Vetiver	3 drops
Carrier Oil	1 tablespoon (15 ml)

Marjoram	4 drops
Mandarin	4 drops
Celery	4 drops
Vanilla (CO_2)	3 drops
Carrier Oil	1 tablespoon (15 ml)

Galbanum	4 drops
Vanilla (CO_2)	4 drops
Amyris	4 drops
Neroli	3 drops
Carrier Oil	1 tablespoon (15 ml)

Champaca Flower	5 drops
Mandarin	5 drops
Spikenard	5 drops
Carrier Oil	1 tablespoon (15 ml)

Spruce	4 drops
Fir Needles	4 drops
Amyris	4 drops
Mandarin	3 drops
Carrier Oil	1 tablespoon (15 ml)

SOUND SLEEP

These formulas can help a person get a better night's sleep. Massage one of these formulas into the middle and lower back, abdomen, and upper chest, for about 30 minutes before bedtime and until the oil is fully absorbed into the skin. After the massage, dab on cornstarch to dry off any remaining oil.

Please note: Due to the relaxing effect of the *Sound Sleep* formulas, a person should not drive a vehicle after receiving the massage.

Tangerine	4 drops
Amyris	4 drops
Marjoram	4 drops
Allspice Berry	2 drops
Spikenard	1 drop
Carrier Oil	1 tablespoon (15 ml)

Marjoram	4 drops
Galbanum	3 drops
Myrtle	3 drops
Petitgrain	3 drops
Anise	2 drops
Carrier Oil	1 tablespoon (15 ml)

Orange	5 drops
Marjoram	4 drops
Champaca Flower	3 drops
Vetiver	3 drops
Carrier Oil	1 tablespoon (15 ml)

Dill	4 drops
Vetiver	4 drops
Guaiacwood	3 drops
Neroli	2 drops
Chamomile (Roman)	2 drops
Carrier Oil	1 tablespoon (15 ml)

Vetiver	4 drops
Amyris	3 drops
Tangerine	3 drops
Clary Sage	3 drops
Lavender	2 drops
Carrier Oil	1 tablespoon (15 ml)

Neroli	4 drops
Mandarin	4 drops
Allspice Berry	3 drops
Rosewood	2 drops
Spruce	2 drops
Carrier Oil	1 tablespoon (15 ml)

Amyris	3 drops
Champaca Flower	3 drops
Anise	3 drops
Spruce	3 drops
Vanilla (CO_2)	3 drops
Carrier Oil	1 tablespoon (15 ml)

Marjoram	4 drops
Cedarwood (Atlas)	3 drops
Clary Sage	3 drops
Vanilla (CO_2)	3 drops
Palmarosa	2 drops
Carrier Oil	1 tablespoon (15 ml)

STRESS-FREE FEET

These formulas soothe and relax the feet as well as assist in getting a restful sleep. Use before going to bed.

Fill a basin with water as warm as you like, add 1/2 cup (4 ounces or 113.4 grams) of Epsom salt (magnesium sulfate), and soak the feet for 15 minutes or longer. Wipe dry, and massage one of the formulas into the bottoms of the feet, ankles, and calves for about 15 minutes on each foot and until the oil is fully absorbed into the skin. After the massage, dab on cornstarch to dry off any remaining oil.

Please note: Due to the relaxing effect of the *Stress-Free Feet* formulas, a person should not drive a vehicle after receiving the massage.

Mandarin	5 drops
Marjoram	4 drops
Dill	4 drops
Vetiver	2 drops
Carrier Oil	1 tablespoon (15 ml)

Dill	4 drops
Grapefruit	4 drops
Spikenard	4 drops
Vanilla (CO_2)	3 drops
Carrier Oil	1 tablespoon (15 ml)

Petitgrain	4 drops
Tangerine	4 drops
Vanilla (CO_2)	4 drops
Cumin	3 drops
Carrier Oil	1 tablespoon (15 ml)

Myrtle	5 drops
Lemon	4 drops
Spruce	4 drops
Cedarwood (Atlas)	2 drops
Carrier Oil	1 tablespoon (15 ml)

Spruce	4 drops
Dill	4 drops
Tangerine	4 drops
Marjoram	3 drops
Carrier Oil	1 tablespoon (15 ml)

Tangerine	4 drops
Dill	4 drops
Petitgrain	4 drops
Spikenard	3 drops
Carrier Oil	1 tablespoon (15 ml)

Amyris	5 drops
Marjoram	4 drops
Orange	3 drops
Eucalyptus Citriodora	3 drops
Carrier Oil	1 tablespoon (15 ml)

Galbanum	4 drops
Neroli	4 drops
Mandarin	4 drops
Grapefruit	3 drops
Carrier Oil	1 tablespoon (15 ml)

Lavender	5 drops
Clary Sage	4 drops
Vanilla (CO_2)	4 drops
Dill	2 drops
Carrier Oil	1 tablespoon (15 ml)

Mandarin	5 drops
Spruce	4 drops
Dill	3 drops
Amyris	3 drops
Carrier Oil	1 tablespoon (15 ml)

Marjoram	4 drops
Rosewood	4 drops
Amyris	4 drops
Ylang-Ylang	3 drops
Carrier Oil	1 tablespoon (15 ml)

Marjoram	4 drops
Eucalyptus Citriodora	4 drops
Fir Needles	4 drops
Allspice Berry	3 drops
Carrier Oil	1 tablespoon (15 ml)

THINK MORE CLEARLY

Massage one of these formulas into the back of the neck, shoulders, back, and upper chest for at least 30 minutes and until the oil is fully absorbed into the skin. After the massage, dab on cornstarch to dry off any remaining oil.

Spruce	5 drops
Myrtle	4 drops
Litsea Cubeba	3 drops
Grapefruit	3 drops
Carrier Oil	1 tablespoon (15 ml)

Fir Needles	4 drops
Spearmint	4 drops
Tangerine	3 drops
Lemon Myrtle	2 drops
Eucalyptus Citriodora	2 drops
Carrier Oil	1 tablespoon (15 ml)

Citronella	3 drops
Spruce	3 drops
Helichrysum	3 drops
Lime	3 drops
Myrtle	3 drops
Carrier Oil	1 tablespoon (15 ml)

Helichrysum	4 drops
Peppermint	4 drops
Allspice Berry	3 drops
Litsea Cubeba	3 drops
Tangerine	1 drop
Carrier Oil	1 tablespoon (15 ml)

Myrtle	4 drops
Spearmint	4 drops
Spruce	4 drops
Thyme	3 drops
Carrier Oil	1 tablespoon (15 ml)

Cabreuva	4 drops
Spearmint	4 drops
Litsea Cubeba	4 drops
Thyme	3 drops
Carrier Oil	1 tablespoon (15 ml)

TUMMY RUB

Massage one of these formulas into the abdominal area for at least 30 minutes and until the oil is fully absorbed into the skin. After the massage, dab on cornstarch to dry off any remaining oil.

Copaiba	4 drops
Helichrysum	3 drops
Lemongrass	3 drops
Peppermint	3 drops
Galbanum	2 drops
Carrier Oil	1 tablespoon (15 ml)

Lemon	4 drops
Mandarin	4 drops
Spearmint	4 drops
Sandalwood	3 drops
Carrier Oil	1 tablespoon (15 ml)

Mandarin	5 drops
Marjoram	4 drops
Litsea Cubeba	4 drops
Ginger	2 drops
Carrier Oil	1 tablespoon (15 ml)

Spearmint	4 drops
Chamomile (Roman)	4 drops
Fennel (Sweet)	3 drops
Patchouli	2 drops
Cabreuva	2 drops
Carrier Oil	1 tablespoon (15 ml)

Helichrysum	4 drops
Fennel (Sweet)	3 drops
Clary Sage	3 drops
Spearmint	3 drops
Patchouli	2 drops
Carrier Oil	1 tablespoon (15 ml)

Lemon	5 drops
Ginger	3 drops
Spearmint	3 drops
Patchouli	3 drops
Tangerine	1 drop
Carrier Oil	1 tablespoon (15 ml)

Mandarin	4 drops
Copaiba	3 drops
Spearmint	3 drops
Litsea Cubeba	3 drops
Fennel (Sweet)	2 drops
Carrier Oil	1 tablespoon (15 ml)

Chamomile (Roman)	4 drops
Vetiver	3 drops
Sage (Spanish)	3 drops
Peppermint	3 drops
Allspice Berry	2 drops
Carrier Oil	1 tablespoon (15 ml)

WARM CIRCULATION

To encourage a feeling of warmth, massage one of these formulas into the back of the neck, shoulders, back, upper chest, abdomen, hands, and feet for at least 30 minutes and until the oil is fully absorbed into the skin. After the massage, dab on cornstarch to dry off any remaining oil.

Thyme	4 drops
Marjoram	4 drops
Allspice Berry	4 drops
Sandalwood	3 drops
Carrier Oil	1 tablespoon (15 ml)

Allspice Berry	4 drops
Copaiba	4 drops
Fennel (Sweet)	3 drops
Cajeput	2 drops
Sandalwood	2 drops
Carrier Oil	1 tablespoon (15 ml)

Cardamom	4 drops
Thyme	4 drops
Copaiba	4 drops
Vetiver	3 drops
Carrier Oil	1 tablespoon (15 ml)

Copaiba	5 drops
Allspice Berry	4 drops
Marjoram	3 drops
Champaca Flower	3 drops
Carrier Oil	1 tablespoon (15 ml)

Cardamom	4 drops
Marjoram	4 drops
Amyris	4 drops
Fennel (Sweet)	3 drops
Carrier Oil	1 tablespoon (15 ml)

Fennel (Sweet)	3 drops
Cinnamon Leaf	3 drops
Cumin	3 drops
Cedarwood (Atlas)	3 drops
Marjoram	3 drops
Carrier Oil	1 tablespoon (15 ml)

Marjoram	4 drops
Allspice Berry	3 drops
Copaiba	3 drops
Fennel (Sweet)	3 drops
Cinnamon Leaf	2 drops
Carrier Oil	1 tablespoon (15 ml)

Marjoram	4 drops
Black Pepper	3 drops
Allspice Berry	3 drops
Ginger	3 drops
Fennel (Sweet)	2 drops
Carrier Oil	1 tablespoon (15 ml)

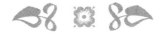

CHAPTER 7

Stress-Less Living

Stress is the body's response when life's demands become overwhelming. It is especially produced on occasions when we suppress our natural instincts or withhold our feelings. If the stressed state is allowed to linger, it causes considerable damage to the body. The adrenal glands can become exhausted, resulting in impaired physical and mental functioning, reduced energy levels, fatigue, and depression. Extended stress may be responsible for an increase in blood pressure, immune-system suppression, heart disease, and other organ and nervous system disorders.

One of the great paradoxes is that with the advancement of modern technology—intended to make life easier—stress-related illnesses keep rising. It has been estimated that as many as 75 percent of all medical complaints are stress related.

> *Use this deep breathing exercise for the formulas in this chapter:*
>
> **Inhale counting slowly from 1 to 6. Hold the breath for a count of 1 to 4, then exhale counting slowly from 1 to 6. Do this exercise for about 10 breaths or more.**

DEEP BREATHING FOR LESS STRESS

Breathing is the foundation of life. However, in most large cities the air pollution from industry and vehicle emissions is so great that it discourages people from breathing deeply. In addition, stress has the same effect, causing a person to breathe shallowly. Deep breathing is essential to relieve stress and maintain good health and well-being. By using essential oils and practicing deep breathing exercises daily, you should notice favorable results.

Deep Breathing for Less Stress—Application

Apply one of these formulas to the upper chest and abdomen until the oil is fully absorbed into the skin. Rub a small amount of the formula on the wrist. During the application, bring the wrist close to the nose and breathe the vapors in deeply. When done, if you wish, dab on cornstarch to dry off any remaining oil.

Eucalyptus Radiata	4 drops
Lemon	4 drops
Amyris	2 drops
Carrier Oil	2 teaspoons (10 ml)

Lavender	4 drops
Spruce	3 drops
Myrtle	3 drops
Carrier Oil	2 teaspoons (10 ml)

Cabreuva	4 drops
Copaiba	3 drops
Lavender	3 drops
Carrier Oil	2 teaspoons (10 ml)

Lavender	3 drops
Marjoram	3 drops
Cabreuva	2 drops
Eucalyptus Radiata	2 drops
Carrier Oil	2 teaspoons (10 ml)

Fir Needles	4 drops
Cajeput	4 drops
Cedarwood (Atlas)	2 drops
Carrier Oil	2 teaspoons (10 ml)

Hyssop Decumbens	4 drops
Cabreuva	4 drops
Cedarwood (Atlas)	2 drops
Carrier Oil	2 teaspoons (10 ml)

Spruce	3 drops
Myrtle	3 drops
Spearmint	2 drops
Lemon	2 drops
Carrier Oil	2 teaspoons (10 ml)

Cabreuva	4 drops
Lavender	4 drops
Cajeput	2 drops
Carrier Oil	2 teaspoons (10 ml)

Marjoram	5 drops
Frankincense	3 drops
Cedarwood (Atlas)	2 drops
Carrier Oil	2 teaspoons (10 ml)

Fir Needles	4 drops
Eucalyptus Citriodora	3 drops
Marjoram	3 drops
Carrier Oil	2 teaspoons (10 ml)

Marjoram	4 drops
Spruce	2 drops
Frankincense	2 drops
Lavender	2 drops
Carrier Oil	2 teaspoons (10 ml)

Eucalyptus Radiata	4 drops
Spruce	3 drops
Ravensara Aromatica	3 drops
Carrier Oil	2 teaspoons (10 ml)

Deep Breathing for Less Stress—Diffuser

Choose one of these formulas. Depending on the type of diffuser you have, place the essential oils in the designated area, then turn on the unit to disperse the aroma into the air.

Mandarin	50%
Lemon	50%

Tangerine	50%
Litsea Cubeba	30%
Spruce	20%

Spruce	100%

Fir Needles	50%
Mandarin	50%

Deep Breathing for Less Stress—Inhaler

Choose one of these formulas. Combine the essential oils in a small glass bottle with a wide opening. Inhale the vapors slowly and deeply. Then tightly cap the bottle after using.

Spruce	25 drops
Frankincense	10 drops

Marjoram	20 drops
Myrtle	10 drops

Frankincense	20 drops
Mandarin	10 drops

Cedarwood (Atlas)	18 drops
Lemon	17 drops

Lavender	15 drops
Litsea Cubeba	10 drops

Spruce	15 drops
Lemon	15 drops
Myrtle	15 drops

Deep Breathing for Less Stress— Mist Spray

Choose one of these formulas. Fill a fine-mist spray bottle with 2 ounces (60 ml) of purified water, then add the essential oils. Tighten the cap and shake well. Mist numerous times over the head with eyes closed. Breathe the vapors in slowly and deeply.

Lavender	25 drops
Cajeput	25 drops
Lemon	25 drops
Pure Water	2 ounces (60 ml)

Eucalyptus Radiata	20 drops
Spruce	20 drops
Lemon	20 drops
Lavender	15 drops
Pure Water	2 ounces (60 ml)

Lavender	35 drops
Frankincense	25 drops
Marjoram	15 drops
Pure Water	2 ounces (60 ml)

Cypress	20 drops
Spearmint	20 drops
Litsea Cubeba	20 drops
Myrtle	15 drops
Pure Water	2 ounces (60 ml)

Eucalyptus Radiata	20 drops
Lavender	20 drops
Spearmint	20 drops
Litsea Cubeba	15 drops
Pure Water	2 ounces (60 ml)

Lemon	20 drops
Spruce	20 drops
Ravensara Aromatica	15 drops
Fir Needles	10 drops
Cedarwood (Atlas)	10 drops
Pure Water	2 ounces (60 ml)

Lavender	23 drops
Lemon	22 drops
Myrtle	15 drops
Marjoram	15 drops
Pure Water	2 ounces (60 ml)

Eucalyptus Radiata	20 drops
Lemon	20 drops
Myrtle	20 drops
Peppermint	15 drops
Pure Water	2 ounces (60 ml)

Lavender	25 drops
Cedarwood (Atlas)	25 drops
Fir Needles	15 drops
Myrtle	10 drops
Pure Water	2 ounces (60 ml)

Marjoram	25 drops
Cajeput	25 drops
Spruce	25 drops
Pure Water	2 ounces (60 ml)

LOWER BACK STRESS RELIEF

It is common for people to experience stress in the lower back. These application formulas can help.

Lower Back Stress Relief—Application

Apply one of these formulas to the lower back until the oil is fully absorbed into the skin. Rub a small amount of the formula on the wrist. During the application, bring the wrist close to the nose and breathe the vapors in deeply. When done, if you wish, dab on cornstarch to dry off any remaining oil.

Helichrysum	4 drops
Marjoram	3 drops
Amyris	3 drops
Carrier Oil	2 teaspoons (10 ml)

Palmarosa	3 drops
Thyme	3 drops
Frankincense	2 drops
Amyris	2 drops
Carrier Oil	2 teaspoons (10 ml)

Helichrysum	4 drops
Thyme	3 drops
Cumin	3 drops
Carrier Oil	2 teaspoons (10 ml)

Geranium	3 drops
Ginger	3 drops
Spikenard	2 drops
Marjoram	2 drops
Carrier Oil	2 teaspoons (10 ml)

Vetiver	3 drops
Celery	3 drops
Cumin	2 drops
Geranium	2 drops
Carrier Oil	2 teaspoons (10 ml)

Thyme	3 drops
Marjoram	3 drops
Helichrysum	2 drops
Ylang-Ylang	2 drops
Carrier Oil	2 teaspoons (10 ml)

Allspice Berry	3 drops
Marjoram	3 drops
Cardamom	2 drops
Frankincense	2 drops
Carrier Oil	2 teaspoons (10 ml)

Allspice Berry	4 drops
Rosewood	3 drops
Amyris	3 drops
Carrier Oil	2 teaspoons (10 ml)

Allspice Berry	4 drops
Manuka	4 drops
Vetiver	2 drops
Carrier Oil	2 teaspoons (10 ml)

Marjoram	3 drops
Manuka	3 drops
Thyme	2 drops
Amyris	2 drops
Carrier Oil	2 teaspoons (10 ml)

Helichrysum	3 drops
Allspice Berry	3 drops
Amyris	2 drops
Cabreuva	2 drops
Carrier Oil	2 teaspoons (10 ml)

Rosewood	3 drops
Amyris	3 drops
Cumin	2 drops
Marjoram	2 drops
Carrier Oil	2 teaspoons (10 ml)

MOTION COMFORT

Some people experience discomfort while traveling. These application and inhaler formulas can help.

Motion Comfort—Application

Choose a formula, apply it on the abdominal area and massage it in well until the oil is fully absorbed into the skin. Rub a small amount of the formula on the wrist. During the application, bring the wrist close to the nose and breathe the vapors in deeply. When done, if you wish, dab on cornstarch to dry off any remaining oil.

Peppermint	4 drops
Cedarwood (Atlas)	3 drops
Litsea Cubeba	3 drops
Carrier Oil	2 teaspoons (10 ml)

Lavender	4 drops
Myrtle	4 drops
Amyris	2 drops
Carrier Oil	2 teaspoons (10 ml)

Allspice Berry	3 drops
Lemon	3 drops
Litsea Cubeba	2 drops
Cedarwood (Atlas)	2 drops
Carrier Oil	2 teaspoons (10 ml)

Peppermint	2 drops
Dill	2 drops
Lavender	2 drops
Litsea Cubeba	2 drops
Cedarwood (Atlas)	2 drops
Carrier Oil	2 teaspoons (10 ml)

Tangerine	3 drops
Litsea Cubeba	3 drops
Spearmint	3 drops
Cedarwood (Atlas)	1 drop
Carrier Oil	2 teaspoons (10 ml)

Fennel	2 drops
Dill	2 drops
Spearmint	2 drops
Lemon	2 drops
Cedarwood (Atlas)	2 drops
Carrier Oil	2 teaspoons (10 ml)

Spearmint	4 drops
Allspice Berry	3 drops
Amyris	3 drops
Carrier Oil	2 teaspoons (10 ml)

Lavender	3 drops
Spearmint	3 drops
Allspice Berry	2 drops
Ginger	2 drops
Carrier Oil	2 teaspoons (10 ml)

Motion Comfort—Inhaler

Choose one of these formulas. Combine the essential oils in a small glass bottle with a wide opening. Inhale the vapors slowly and deeply. Then tightly cap the bottle after using.

Spearmint	15 drops
Amyris	5 drops

Allspice Berry	10 drops
Peppermint	10 drops

Litsea Cubeba	10 drops
Allspice Berry	5 drops
Cedarwood (Atlas)	5 drops

Lavender	8 drops
Peppermint	7 drops
Amyris	5 drops

Peppermint	20 drops

Chamomile (Roman)	10 drops
Spearmint	10 drops

Chamomile (Roman)	10 drops
Lavender	10 drops

Spearmint	15 drops
Allspice Berry	5 drops

PEACE & CALM

There are times when a person may want to be alone in a quiet atmosphere to comfort an overly stressed nervous system.

Find a quiet, comfortable place to relax where you will not be disturbed, use one of the formulas, and enjoy the peacefulness.

Peace & Calm—Application

Apply one of these formulas to the upper chest and back of the neck, until the oil is fully absorbed into the skin. Rub a small amount of the formula on the wrist. During the application, bring the wrist close to the nose and breathe the vapors in deeply. When done, if you wish, dab on cornstarch to dry off any remaining oil.

Chamomile (Roman)	4 drops
Tangerine	4 drops
Vetiver	2 drops
Carrier Oil	2 teaspoons (10 ml)

Neroli	4 drops
Tangerine	4 drops
Sandalwood	2 drops
Carrier Oil	2 teaspoons (10 ml)

Mandarin	4 drops
Petitgrain	3 drops
Amyris	3 drops
Carrier Oil	2 teaspoons (10 ml)

Lavender	4 drops
Spikenard	3 drops
Orange	3 drops
Carrier Oil	2 teaspoons (10 ml)

Vetiver	4 drops
Ylang-Ylang	3 drops
Bergamot	3 drops
Carrier Oil	2 teaspoons (10 ml)

Neroli	4 drops
Cabreuva	3 drops
Spikenard	3 drops
Carrier Oil	2 teaspoons (10 ml)

Peace & Calm—Inhaler

Choose one of these formulas. Combine the essential oils in a small glass bottle with a wide opening. Inhale the vapors slowly and deeply. Then tightly cap the bottle after using.

Tangerine	15 drops
Neroli	8 drops

Spruce	15 drops
Lemon	10 drops

Orange	25 drops
Marjoram	10 drops

Orange	25 drops
Lavender	10 drops
Vanilla (CO_2)	5 drops

Peace & Calm—Mist Spray

Choose one of these formulas. Fill a fine-mist spray bottle with 2 ounces (60 ml) of purified water, then add the essential oils. Tighten the cap and shake well. Mist numerous times over the head with eyes closed. Breathe the vapors in slowly and deeply.

Orange	25 drops
Petitgrain	25 drops
Lemon	15 drops
Amyris	10 drops
Pure Water	2 ounces (60 ml)

Tangerine	20 drops
Spruce	20 drops
Dill	18 drops
Spikenard	17 drops
Pure Water	2 ounces (60 ml)

Rosewood	25 drops
Mandarin	20 drops
Lemon	20 drops
Cedarwood (Atlas)	10 drops
Pure Water	2 ounces (60 ml)

Lemon	25 drops
Basil (Sweet)	15 drops
Ylang-Ylang	15 drops
Amyris	10 drops
Rosewood	10 drops
Pure Water	2 ounces (60 ml)

RELAX THE LEGS

Some people have a problem keeping their legs still. These application formulas should help when used regularly.

Relax the Legs—Application

Before bedtime, fill a basin with water, as warm as you can take, and add 1 cup (8 ounces or 225 grams) of Epsom salt (magnesium sulfate). Soak your feet for 15 to 30 minutes. Wipe dry and apply one of these formulas on the bottoms of the feet, ankles, and calves. Massage in until the oil is fully absorbed into the skin. Rub a small amount of the formula on the wrist. During the application, bring the wrist close to the nose and breathe the vapors in deeply. When done, dab on cornstarch to fully dry off any remaining oil.

Lavender	5 drops
Spruce	5 drops
Vetiver	5 drops
Carrier Oil	1 tablespoon (15 ml)

Marjoram	5 drops
Vetiver	5 drops
Orange	5 drops
Carrier Oil	1 tablespoon (15 ml)

Rosewood	5 drops
Marjoram	5 drops
Amyris	3 drops
Lemon	2 drops
Carrier Oil	1 tablespoon (15 ml)

Marjoram	4 drops
Vanilla (CO_2)	4 drops
Dill	3 drops
Celery	2 drops
Amyris	2 drops
Carrier Oil	1 tablespoon (15 ml)

Myrtle	4 drops
Tangerine	4 drops
Marjoram	3 drops
Amyris	2 drops
Cedarwood (Atlas)	2 drops
Carrier Oil	1 tablespoon (15 ml)

Lavender	4 drops
Vetiver	4 drops
Galbanum	4 drops
Marjoram	3 drops
Carrier Oil	1 tablespoon (15 ml)

Celery	3 drops
Rosewood	3 drops
Vanilla (CO_2)	3 drops
Mandarin	3 drops
Dill	3 drops
Carrier Oil	1 tablespoon (15 ml)

Dill	4 drops
Marjoram	4 drops
Vetiver	4 drops
Vanilla (CO_2)	3 drops
Carrier Oil	1 tablespoon (15 ml)

Dill	4 drops
Orange	4 drops
Vanilla (CO_2)	4 drops
Galbanum	3 drops
Carrier Oil	1 tablespoon (15 ml)

Allspice Berry	4 drops
Marjoram	4 drops
Mandarin	4 drops
Vetiver	3 drops
Carrier Oil	1 tablespoon (15 ml)

Rosewood	4 drops
Marjoram	4 drops
Vanilla (CO_2)	4 drops
Ylang-Ylang	2 drops
Lemon Myrtle	1 drop
Carrier Oil	1 tablespoon (15 ml)

Tangerine	4 drops
Cabreuva	4 drops
Amyris	4 drops
Rosewood	3 drops
Carrier Oil	1 tablespoon (15 ml)

SLEEP PEACEFULLY

High levels of stress and the inability to get a restful sleep can cause a vicious cycle. If you are highly stressed, it is difficult to get a good night's rest—and if you don't get a good night's rest, you're likely to develop more stress.

According to estimates, about 17 percent of the population has difficulty sleeping. Some have problems falling asleep, while others wake up and have difficulty returning to sleep.

Helpful Tips for Better Sleep

- Don't eat for at least three hours before bed-time.

- Avoid excitement before going to sleep.

- Make sure your bedroom is clean and neat.

- Use natural fibers for bed linens, covers, and nightwear.

- Do deep breathing exercises using essential oils (pages 107–110).

- Receive a relaxing massage with essential oils before going to bed.

Sleep Peacefully—Application

Right before going to sleep, apply one of these formulas to the upper chest and back of the neck, until the oil is fully absorbed into the skin. Rub a small amount of the formula on the wrist. During the application, bring the wrist close to the nose and breathe the vapors in deeply. When done, if you wish, dab on cornstarch to dry off any remaining oil.

Marjoram	4 drops
Mandarin	3 drops
Spikenard	3 drops
Carrier Oil	2 teaspoons (10 ml)

Mandarin	5 drops
Neroli	3 drops
Spikenard	2 drops
Carrier Oil	2 teaspoons (10 ml)

Dill	4 drops
Neroli	3 drops
Vetiver	3 drops
Carrier Oil	2 teaspoons (10 ml)

Mandarin	4 drops
Chamomile (Roman)	3 drops
Vetiver	3 drops
Carrier Oil	2 teaspoons (10 ml)

Chamomile (Roman)	4 drops
Marjoram	3 drops
Neroli	3 drops
Carrier Oil	2 teaspoons (10 ml)

Celery	4 drops
Mandarin	3 drops
Amyris	3 drops
Carrier Oil	2 teaspoons (10 ml)

Ylang-Ylang	4 drops
Celery	3 drops
Spikenard	3 drops
Carrier Oil	2 teaspoons (10 ml)

Marjoram	3 drops
Frankincense	3 drops
Cumin	2 drops
Amyris	2 drops
Carrier Oil	2 teaspoons (10 ml)

Spikenard	3 drops
Mandarin	3 drops
Frankincense	2 drops
Spruce	2 drops
Carrier Oil	2 teaspoons (10 ml)

Vanilla (CO_2)	3 drops
Chamomile (Roman)	3 drops
Bergamot	2 drops
Vetiver	2 drops
Carrier Oil	2 teaspoons (10 ml)

Mandarin	4 drops
Vetiver	3 drops
Marjoram	3 drops
Carrier Oil	2 teaspoons (10 ml)

Amyris	4 drops
Marjoram	3 drops
Spikenard	3 drops
Carrier Oil	2 teaspoons (10 ml)

Sleep Peacefully—Mist Spray

Choose one of these formulas. Fill a fine-mist spray bottle with 2 ounces (60 ml) of purified water, then add the essential oils. Tighten the cap and shake well. Mist numerous times over the head with eyes closed. Breathe the vapors in slowly and deeply.

Lavender	20 drops
Celery	15 drops
Marjoram	15 drops
Copaiba	15 drops
Litsea Cubeba	10 drops
Pure Water	2 ounces (60 ml)

Tangerine	30 drops
Marjoram	15 drops
Neroli	10 drops
Amyris	10 drops
Celery	10 drops
Pure Water	2 ounces (60 ml)

Celery	20 drops
Tangerine	20 drops
Amyris	20 drops
Marjoram	15 drops
Pure Water	2 ounces (60 ml)

Dill	25 drops
Marjoram	25 drops
Lavender	15 drops
Vanilla (CO_2)	10 drops
Pure Water	2 ounces (60 ml)

SOLAR PLEXUS (ABDOMINAL) DE-STRESSOR

Many people store their stress in the abdominal area. These application formulas can help to ease some of the stress.

Solar Plexus (Abdominal) De-Stressor— Application

Apply one of these formulas to the abdominal area until the oil is fully absorbed into the skin. Rub a small amount of the formula on the wrist. During the application, bring the wrist close to the nose and breathe the vapors in deeply. When done, if you wish, dab on cornstarch to dry off any remaining oil.

Helichrysum	4 drops
Clary Sage	3 drops
Amyris	3 drops
Carrier Oil	2 teaspoons (10 ml)

Geranium	4 drops
Cypress	3 drops
Neroli	3 drops
Carrier Oil	2 teaspoons (10 ml)

Rosewood	4 drops
Fennel (Sweet)	3 drops
Chamomile (Roman)	3 drops
Carrier Oil	2 teaspoons (10 ml)

Mandarin	3 drops
Marjoram	3 drops
Helichrysum	2 drops
Cumin	2 drops
Carrier Oil	2 teaspoons (10 ml)

Geranium	3 drops
Ginger	3 drops
Amyris	2 drops
Fennel (Sweet)	2 drops
Carrier Oil	2 teaspoons (10 ml)

Lemon	3 drops
Mandarin	3 drops
Dill	2 drops
Neroli	2 drops
Carrier Oil	2 teaspoons (10 ml)

Amyris	4 drops
Marjoram	3 drops
Clary Sage	3 drops
Carrier Oil	2 teaspoons (10 ml)

Neroli	3 drops
Cypress	3 drops
Petitgrain	2 drops
Fennel (Sweet)	2 drops
Carrier Oil	2 teaspoons (10 ml)

Tangerine	3 drops
Chamomile (Roman)	3 drops
Cumin	2 drops
Celery	2 drops
Carrier Oil	2 teaspoons (10 ml)

Neroli	3 drops
Ylang-Ylang	3 drops
Helichrysum	2 drops
Lemon	2 drops
Carrier Oil	2 teaspoons (10 ml)

Lemon	4 drops
Cedarwood (Atlas)	3 drops
Cypress	3 drops
Carrier Oil	2 teaspoons (10 ml)

Mandarin	2 drops
Ginger	2 drops
Dill	2 drops
Amyris	2 drops
Helichrysum	2 drops
Carrier Oil	2 teaspoons (10 ml)

STOP SNORING!

Snoring can cause stress to other people in the house who are kept awake by the noisy snorer. Many married couples have to sleep in separate rooms because one spouse snores. Repeat the application or mist spray formula nightly for best results.

Stop Snoring!—Application

Before going to sleep, apply one of these formulas to the upper chest and back of the neck, until the oil is fully absorbed into the skin. Rub a small amount of the formula on the wrist. During the application, bring the wrist close to the nose and breathe the vapors in deeply. When done, if you wish, dab on cornstarch to dry off any remaining oil.

If snoring occurs during the night, use one of the *Stop Snoring!* mist sprays.

Helichrysum	5 drops
Lavender	5 drops
Carrier Oil	2 teaspoons (10 ml)

Cedarwood (Atlas)	4 drops
Helichrysum	3 drops
Anise	3 drops
Carrier Oil	2 teaspoons (10 ml)

Amyris	4 drops
Lavender	4 drops
Citronella	2 drops
Carrier Oil	2 teaspoons (10 ml)

Litsea Cubeba	3 drops
Marjoram	3 drops
Lavender	2 drops
Spruce	2 drops
Carrier Oil	2 teaspoons (10 ml)

Copaiba	4 drops
Marjoram	4 drops
Cabreuva	2 drops
Carrier Oil	2 teaspoons (10 ml)

Ravensara Aromatica	3 drops
Lavender	3 drops
Cedarwood (Atlas)	2 drops
Spruce	2 drops
Carrier Oil	2 teaspoons (10 ml)

Cedarwood (Atlas)	5 drops
Dill	3 drops
Lemon	2 drops
Carrier Oil	2 teaspoons (10 ml)

Lavender	4 drops
Marjoram	3 drops
Ravensara Aromatica	3 drops
Carrier Oil	2 teaspoons (10 ml)

Marjoram	4 drops
Lemon	3 drops
Hyssop Decumbens	3 drops
Carrier Oil	2 teaspoons (10 ml)

Hyssop Decumbens	4 drops
Cedarwood (Atlas)	3 drops
Mandarin	3 drops
Carrier Oil	2 teaspoons (10 ml)

Stop Snoring!—Mist Spray

Choose one of these formulas. Fill a fine-mist spray bottle with 2 ounces (60 ml) of purified water, add the essential oils, tighten the cap, and shake well. Before bedtime, mist numerous times over the snorer's head and have him or her inhale the vapors slowly and deeply. If the person begins to snore during the night, mist the spray again. Avoid getting the mist near the snorer's eyes. Repeat misting for several nights until best results are obtained.

Lavender	30 drops
Cedarwood (Atlas)	30 drops
Citronella	15 drops
Pure Water	2 ounces (10 ml)

Marjoram	25 drops
Spruce	18 drops
Tangerine	17 drops
Amyris	15 drops
Pure Water	2 ounces (60 ml)

Ravensara Aromatica	25 drops
Marjoram	25 drops
Cedarwood (Atlas)	25 drops
Pure Water	2 ounces (60 ml)

Spruce	20 drops
Copaiba	20 drops
Fir Needles	20 drops
Cedarwood (Atlas)	15 drops
Pure Water	2 ounces (60 ml)

Petitgrain	15 drops
Neroli	15 drops
Lavender	15 drops
Cabreuva	15 drops
Citronella	15 drops
Pure Water	2 ounces (60 ml)

Spruce	25 drops
Petitgrain	20 drops
Lavender	15 drops
Marjoram	10 drops
Pine	5 drops
Pure Water	2 ounces (60 ml)

Mandarin	25 drops
Amyris	25 drops
Spruce	15 drops
Hyssop Decumbens	10 drops
Pure Water	2 ounces (60 ml)

Hyssop Decumbens	20 drops
Cedarwood (Atlas)	20 drops
Tangerine	20 drops
Marjoram	15 drops
Pure Water	2 ounces (60 ml)

Cedarwood (Atlas)	25 drops
Dill	20 drops
Bergamot	15 drops
Lavender	15 drops
Pure Water	2 ounces (60 ml)

Amyris	25 drops
Marjoram	25 drops
Spruce	15 drops
Lemon	10 drops
Pure Water	2 ounces (60 ml)

Amyris	20 drops
Dill	20 drops
Mandarin	20 drops
Fir Needles	15 drops
Pure Water	2 ounces (60 ml)

Cajeput	20 drops
Lavender	20 drops
Cedarwood (Atlas)	20 drops
Mandarin	15 drops
Pure Water	2 ounces (60 ml)

YOGA & EXERCISE

Yoga exercises have become popular in the West in recent years. The deep breathing and stretching exercises are an excellent way to increase flexibility, strengthen the body, and reduce stress.

Yoga & Exercise—Application

Apply one of these formulas on the muscles and joints you want to stretch prior to doing the exercise. Massage in well until the oil is fully absorbed into the skin. Rub a small amount of the formula on the wrist. During the application, bring the wrist close to the nose and breathe the vapors in deeply. When done, if you wish, dab on cornstarch to dry off any remaining oil.

Lemon	4 drops
Thyme	4 drops
Cedarwood (Atlas)	2 drops
Carrier Oil	2 teaspoons (10 ml)

Geranium	4 drops
Rosewood	3 drops
Sandalwood	3 drops
Carrier Oil	2 teaspoons (10 ml)

Cedarwood (Atlas)	4 drops
Cinnamon Leaf	3 drops
Orange	2 drops
Black Pepper	1 drop
Carrier Oil	2 teaspoons (10 ml)

Marjoram	3 drops
Helichrysum	3 drops
Allspice Berry	3 drops
Amyris	1 drop
Carrier Oil	2 teaspoons (10 ml)

Geranium	3 drops
Orange	3 drops
Rosewood	3 drops
Amyris	1 drop
Carrier Oil	2 teaspoons (10 ml)

Tangerine	4 drops
Thyme	4 drops
Amyris	2 drops
Carrier Oil	2 teaspoons (10 ml)

Helichrysum	4 drops
Cinnamon Leaf	3 drops
Litsea Cubeba	2 drops
Ylang-Ylang	1 drop
Carrier Oil	2 teaspoons (10 ml)

Cedarwood (Atlas)	3 drops
Thyme	3 drops
Cabreuva	2 drops
Ylang-Ylang	2 drops
Carrier Oil	2 teaspoons (10 ml)

Helichrysum	4 drops
Ylang-Ylang	4 drops
Vetiver	2 drops
Carrier Oil	2 teaspoons (10 ml)

Allspice Berry	3 drops
Ylang-Ylang	3 drops
Galbanum	2 drops
Lemon	2 drops
Carrier Oil	2 teaspoons (10 ml)

Helichrysum	4 drops
Juniper Berry	3 drops
Thyme	3 drops
Carrier Oil	2 teaspoons (10 ml)

Vetiver	4 drops
Lemon	2 drops
Helichrysum	2 drops
Cumin	2 drops
Carrier Oil	2 teaspoons (10 ml)

CHAPTER 8

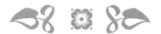

Personal Care, Health, and Home

Over the past fifty years our dependency on the use of chemicals as ingredients in products has proliferated in practically every facet of our life. It is commonplace today for a person to be exposed to thousands of chemicals daily—some very harmful to health.

It is becoming more obvious to many people that we must take greater responsibility for our actions and use products that are compatible with our natural environment. Our earth is a sacred embodiment that makes all life possible. We have an obligation to preserve and maintain her integrity not only for the benefit of our future but for future generations as well.

It is easy and so enjoyable to produce your own natural everyday products to improve the quality of life and, at the same time, be considerate and caring for the environment. It takes minutes to mix all the ingredients together and use. You'll derive great satisfaction knowing that you made these products yourself!

BATH OILS

Besides being necessary for hygiene, baths are beneficial for good health.

Soaking in warm water scented with essential oils can be so pleasurable that once you experience an aromatic bath, plain water baths will become a thing of the past. These formulas will also help moisturize the skin.

Choose one of these formulas. Mix the essential oils and carrier oil together in a small glass bottle. Close the bathroom window and door. Fill the bathtub with water, as warm as you like. Then pour the bath-oil formula into the bathwater. Swirl the water to distribute the oils evenly throughout the tub. Enter the bath immediately to capture all the benefits of the essential oils. Relax and enjoy your bath for 30 minutes.

Calming—Bath Oil

Spruce	5 drops
Frankincense	5 drops
Marjoram	3 drops
Mandarin	2 drops
Carrier Oil	1 teaspoon (5 ml)

Ylang-Ylang	4 drops
Cabreuva	4 drops
Petitgrain	4 drops
Cedarwood (Atlas)	3 drops
Carrier Oil	1 teaspoon (5 ml)

Chamomile (Roman)	5 drops
Dill	5 drops
Lemon	3 drops
Guaiacwood	2 drops
Carrier Oil	1 teaspoon (5 ml)

Champaca Flower	4 drops
Dill	4 drops
Amyris	4 drops
Mandarin	3 drops
Carrier Oil	1 teaspoon (5 ml)

Rejuvenating—Bath Oil

Helichrysum	5 drops
Cabreuva	4 drops
Rosemary	4 drops
Spearmint	2 drops
Carrier Oil	1 teaspoon (5 ml)

Eucalyptus Radiata	4 drops
Ravensara Aromatica	4 drops
Lemon	3 drops
Spearmint	3 drops
Rosemary	1 drop
Carrier Oil	1 teaspoon (5 ml)

Rosemary	5 drops
Eucalyptus Citriodora	5 drops
Fir Needles	5 drops
Carrier Oil	1 teaspoon (5 ml)

Helichrysum	4 drops
Eucalyputs Citriodora	4 drops
Patchouli	3 drops
Spearmint	3 drops
Fir Needles	1 drop
Carrier Oil	1 teaspoon (5 ml)

BATH SALTS

Choose one of these formulas. Depending on the bath formula, measure 1 cup (8 ounces or 225 grams) and pour the Epsom salt (magnesium sulfate) or sea salt (fine ground) into a wide-mouthed glass jar, add the essential oils, and mix well. Then place the cap on the jar and tighten. Close the bathroom window and door. Fill the bathtub with water, as warm as you like, and pour the bath-salt formula into the bathwater. Swirl the water to distribute and dissolve the salt to prevent it from settling on the bottom of the tub.

Enter the bath immediately to capture all the benefits of the essential oils. Be careful getting into the tub, since any undissolved salt can make the tub surface slippery. Relax for 30 minutes.

Calming—Bath Salts

Neroli	5 drops
Petitgrain	5 drops
Lemon	3 drops
Mandarin	2 drops
Epsom Salt	1 cup (225 g)

Chamomile (Roman)	5 drops
Lavender	5 drops
Amyris	5 drops
Epsom Salt	1 cup (225 g)

Ylang-Ylang	4 drops
Petitgrain	4 drops
Cedarwood (Atlas)	3 drops
Lemon	3 drops
Dill	1 drop
Epsom Salt	1 cup (225 g)

Neroli	5 drops
Dill	4 drops
Petitgrain	4 drops
Guaiacwood	2 drops
Epsom Salt	1 cup (225 g)

Rejuvenating—Bath Salts

Cypress	5 drops
Rosemary	4 drops
Spearmint	3 drops
Patchouli	3 drops
Sea Salt	1 cup (225 g)

Spruce	4 drops
Eucalyptus Radiata	4 drops
Spearmint	3 drops
Fir Needles	3 drops
Helichrysum	1 drop
Sea Salt	1 cup (225 g)

Fir Needles	5 drops
Rosemary	4 drops
Spruce	4 drops
Patchouli	2 drops
Sea Salt	1 cup (225 g)

Eucalyptus Citriodora	4 drops
Geranium	4 drops
Spearmint	3 drops
Patchouli	3 drops
Helichrysum	1 drop
Sea Salt	1 cup (225 g)

BATHROOM MIST SPRAY FRESHENERS

Choose one of these formulas. Fill a fine-mist spray glass bottle with 2 ounces (60 ml) of purified water, add the essential oils, tighten the cap, and shake well. Mist numerous times in the room to freshen the air. Place a label on the bottle and store in a dark, cool place.

Spearmint	50 drops
Amyris	15 drops
Litsea Cubeba	10 drops
Pure Water	2 ounces (60 ml)

Orange	45 drops
Cinnamon Leaf	20 drops
Cedarwood (Atlas)	10 drops
Pure Water	2 ounces (60 ml)

Eucalyptus Citriodora	40 drops
Grapefruit	20 drops
Patchouli	10 drops
Litsea Cubeba	5 drops
Pure Water	2 ounces (60 ml)

Spruce	40 drops
Fir Needles	15 drops
Pine	10 drops
Cedarwood (Atlas)	10 drops
Pure Water	2 ounces (60 ml)

Spearmint	25 drops
Cedarwood (Atlas)	25 drops
Eucalyptus Citriodora	25 drops
Pure Water	2 ounces (60 ml)

Peppermint	35 drops
Cedarwood (Atlas)	20 drops
Anise	10 drops
Cinnamon Leaf	10 drops
Pure Water	2 ounces (60 ml)

COLDS & FLU: BREATHE FRESH AIR

These formulas can help freshen the air in an indoor environment where someone has a cold or the flu.

Colds & Flu: Breathe Fresh Air— Mist Spray

Choose one of these formulas. Fill a fine-mist spray bottle with 2 ounces (60 ml) of liquid colloidal silver, or distilled water, or a combination of colloidal silver and distilled water. Then add the essential oils. Tighten the cap and shake well. Mist numerous times over the head with eyes closed. Breathe the vapors in slowly and deeply. Place a label on the bottle and store in a dark, cool place.

Please note: Distilled water can be either substituted for the colloidal silver solution or mixed together in any ratio in these formulas to make up the 2 ounces (60 ml). If diluting the colloidal silver, only use distilled water; otherwise water that contains chlorine will render the colloidal silver inactive.

Lemon	25 drops
Manuka	25 drops
Cinnamon Leaf	25 drops
Colloidal Silver Solution and/or Distilled Water	2 ounces (60 ml)

Ravensara Aromatica	20 drops
Cajeput	20 drops
Manuka	20 drops
Bergamot	15 drops
Colloidal Silver Solution and/or Distilled Water	2 ounces (60 ml)

Cinnamon Leaf	20 drops
Ravensara Aromatica	20 drops
Eucalyptus Citriodora	20 drops
Juniper Berry	15 drops
Colloidal Silver Solution and/or Distilled Water	2 ounces (60 ml)

Marjoram	25 drops
Peppermint	25 drops
Cedarwood (Atlas)	15 drops
Juniper Berry	10 drops
Colloidal Silver Solution and/or Distilled Water	2 ounces (60 ml)

Eucalytpus Radiata	35 drops
Lemon	20 drops
Spearmint	10 drops
Cedarwood (Atlas)	10 drops
Colloidal Silver Solution and/or Distilled Water	2 ounces (60 ml)

Thyme	25 drops
Ravensara Aromatica	20 drops
Rosemary	15 drops
Peppermint	15 drops
Colloidal Silver Solution and/or Distilled Water	2 ounces (60 ml)

Thyme	25 drops
Cinnamon Leaf	25 drops
Peppermint	25 drops
Colloidal Silver Solution and/or Distilled Water	2 ounces (60 ml)

Peppermint	25 drops
Rosemary	25 drops
Allspice Berry	25 drops
Colloidal Silver Solution and/or Distilled Water	2 ounces (60 ml)

Cinnamon Leaf	20 drops
Rosemary	20 drops
Clove Bud	20 drops
Spruce	15 drops
Colloidal Silver Solution and/or Distilled Water	2 ounces (60 ml)

Allspice Berry	26 drops
Cinnamon Leaf	19 drops
Fir Needles	15 drops
Lemon	15 drops
Colloidal Silver Solution and/or Distilled Water	2 ounces (60 ml)

Thyme	25 drops
Lemon	20 drops
Tangerine	15 drops
Allspice Berry	15 drops
Colloidal Silver Solution and/or Distilled Water	2 ounces (60 ml)

Clove Bud	20 drops
Rosemary	20 drops
Lemon	20 drops
Manuka	15 drops
Colloidal Silver Solution and/or Distilled Water	2 ounces (60 ml)

CREAMS—BODY CARE

The skin is often taken for granted due to its ability to recover from burns, bruises, cuts, scrapes, and scratches, along with other types of injuries and wounds that are inflicted in the course of our daily life.

Apply a small amount of one of these creams daily to help keep your skin looking younger, healthier and feeling softer.

To prepare the formula, place the shea butter into a small wide-mouthed glass jar. Put the jar in a small pot of water, and warm on a low temperature. When the butter is melted, add the carrier oil, mix well, and remove from the heat. As the mixture cools, add the essential oils, stir well, and cap the jar. Use as needed. Place a label on the jar and store in a dark, cool place.

Please note: If you prefer, you can substitute unrefined sesame seed oil or another carrier oil for evening primrose.

Frankincense	12 drops
Litsea Cubeba	12 drops
Patchouli	6 drops
Vanilla (CO_2)	5 drops
Shea Butter	2 tablespoons (30 ml)
Evening Primrose Oil	8 teaspoons (40 ml)

Copaiba	9 drops
Cedarwood (Atlas)	9 drops
Frankincense	9 drops
Tangerine	8 drops
Shea Butter	2 tablespoons (30 ml)
Evening Primrose Oil	8 teaspoons (40 ml)

Copaiba	15 drops
Lavender	10 drops
Geranium	5 drops
Vanilla (CO_2)	5 drops
Shea Butter	2 tablespoons (30 ml)
Evening Primrose Oil	8 teaspoons (40 ml)

Litsea Cubeba	10 drops
Palmarosa	10 drops
Amyris	10 drops
Geranium	5 drops
Shea Butter	2 tablespoons (30 ml)
Evening Primrose Oil	8 teaspoons (40 ml)

CREAMS—FACIAL CARE

Having healthy looking skin adds to one's beauty. Try one of these creams, and improve the softness and radiance of your skin.

To prepare the formula, place the shea butter into a small wide-mouthed glass jar. Put the jar in a small pot of water, and warm on a low temperature. When the butter is melted, add the carrier oil, mix well, and remove from the heat. As the mixture cools, add the essential oils, stir well, and cap the jar. Use as needed. Place a label on the jar and store in a dark, cool place.

Vanilla (CO_2)	10 drops
Tangerine	10 drops
Cedarwood (Atlas)	10 drops
Shea Butter	2 tablespoons (30 ml)
Jojoba Oil	8 teaspoons (40 ml)

Ylang-Ylang	10 drops
Lemon	8 drops
Cedarwood (Atlas)	7 drops
Petitgrain	5 drops
Shea Butter	2 tablespoons (30 ml)
Jojoba Oil	8 teaspoons (40 ml)

Champaca Flower	10 drops
Amyris	10 drops
Orange	5 drops
Rose	5 drops
Shea Butter	2 tablespoons (30 ml)
Jojoba Oil	8 teaspoons (40 ml)

Vanilla (CO_2)	9 drops
Geranium	9 drops
Sandalwood	8 drops
Lemon	4 drops
Shea Butter	2 tablespoons (30 ml)
Jojoba Oil	8 teaspoons (40 ml)

Palmarosa	13 drops
Rosewood	12 drops
Copaiba	5 drops
Shea Butter	2 tablespoons (30 ml)
Jojoba Oil	8 teaspoons (40 ml)

Vanilla (CO_2)	10 drops
Neroli	10 drops
Palmarosa	10 drops
Shea Butter	2 tablespoons (30 ml)
Jojoba Oil	8 teaspoons (40 ml)

Champaca Flower	12 drops
Chamomile (Roman)	10 drops
Tangerine	8 drops
Shea Butter	2 tablespoons (30 ml)
Jojoba Oil	8 teaspoons (40 ml)

Geranium	10 drops
Rosewood	10 drops
Champaca Flower	10 drops
Shea Butter	2 tablespoons (30 ml)
Jojoba Oil	8 teaspoons (40 ml)

DEEP BREATHING TO REJUVENATE

These formulas will help you breathe more easily and rejuvenate mentally and physically.

Deep Breathing to Rejuvenate— Application

Apply one of these formulas to the upper chest, abdomen, and back of the neck, until the oil is fully absorbed into the skin. Rub a small amount of the formula on the wrist. During the application, bring the wrist close to the nose and breathe the vapors in deeply. When done, if you wish, dab on cornstarch to dry off any remaining oil.

PERSONAL CARE, HEALTH, AND HOME

Peppermint	4 drops
Cedarwood (Atlas)	3 drops
Helichrysum	3 drops
Carrier Oil	2 teaspoons (10 ml)

Rosemary	4 drops
Spruce	3 drops
Helichrysum	3 drops
Carrier Oil	2 teaspoons (10 ml)

Frankincense	4 drops
Spearmint	4 drops
Cedarwood (Atlas)	2 drops
Carrier Oil	2 teaspoons (10 ml)

Spruce	4 drops
Eucalyptus Radiata	3 drops
Helichrysum	3 drops
Carrier Oil	2 teaspoons (10 ml)

Cajeput	4 drops
Helichrysum	3 drops
Lemon	3 drops
Carrier Oil	2 teaspoons (10 ml)

Spearmint	4 drops
Cedarwood (Atlas)	3 drops
Ravensara Aromatica	3 drops
Carrier Oil	2 teaspoons (10 ml)

Eucalyptus Citriodora	4 drops
Cabreuva	3 drops
Peppermint	3 drops
Carrier Oil	2 teaspoons (10 ml)

Helichrysum	4 drops
Spearmint	4 drops
Eucalyptus Citriodora	2 drops
Carrier Oil	2 teaspoons (10 ml)

Spearmint	4 drops
Lemon	4 drops
Rosemary	2 drops
Carrier Oil	2 teaspoons (10 ml)

Cabreuva	4 drops
Litsea Cubeba	3 drops
Eucalyptus Radiata	3 drops
Carrier Oil	2 teaspoons (10 ml)

Deep Breathing to Rejuvenate— Mist Spray

Choose one of these formulas. Fill a fine-mist spray bottle with 2 ounces (60 ml) of purified water, add the essential oils, tighten the cap, and shake well. Mist numerous times over the head with eyes closed. Breathe the vapors in slowly and deeply. Place a label on the bottle and store in a dark, cool place.

Spearmint	20 drops
Helichrysum	20 drops
Amyris	18 drops
Cajeput	17 drops
Pure Water	2 ounces (60 ml)

Frankincense	25 drops
Lemon	20 drops
Cedarwood (Atlas)	15 drops
Myrtle	15 drops
Pure Water	2 ounces (60 ml)

Fir Needles	20 drops
Helichrysum	20 drops
Ravensara Aromatica	20 drops
Lavender	15 drops
Pure Water	2 ounces (60 ml)

127

Peppermint	25 drops
Frankincense	20 drops
Cajeput	15 drops
Eucalyptus Radiata	15 drops
Pure Water	2 ounces (60 ml)

Eucalyptus Radiata	20 drops
Spruce	20 drops
Helichrysum	20 drops
Lime	15 drops
Pure Water	2 ounces (60 ml)

Spearmint	20 drops
Frankincense	20 drops
Helichrysum	20 drops
Amyris	15 drops
Pure Water	2 ounces (60 ml)

Fir Needles	20 drops
Peppermint	20 drops
Amyris	18 drops
Cabreuva	17 drops
Pure Water	2 ounces (60 ml)

Spearmint	25 drops
Fir Needles	15 drops
Helichrysum	15 drops
Rosemary	10 drops
Cedarwood (Atlas)	10 drops
Pure Water	2 ounces (60 ml)

Spearmint	30 drops
Myrtle	20 drops
Cabreuva	15 drops
Amyris	10 drops
Pure Water	2 ounces (60 ml)

Myrtle	20 drops
Litsea Cubeba	20 drops
Ravensara Aromatica	18 drops
Lime	17 drops
Pure Water	2 ounces (60 ml)

DEODORANT POWDERS FOR UNDERARMS & FEET

Choose one of these formulas. Measure 4 tablespoons (2 ounces or 56.7 grams) of cornstarch and pour it into a small wide-mouthed glass jar, add the essential oils, and mix thoroughly. Tighten the cap and let the mixture sit for a day to allow the scent to permeate the powder.

Apply a small portion to the underarms or feet and rub in well. Place a label on the jar and store in a dark, cool place.

Champaca Flower	20 drops
Manuka	20 drops
Vanilla (CO_2)	20 drops
Cornstarch	4 tablespoons (56.7 g)

Manuka	45 drops
Vanilla (CO_2)	15 drops
Cornstarch	4 tablespoons (56.7 g)

Manuka	30 drops
Spikenard	20 drops
Chamomile (Roman)	10 drops
Cornstarch	4 tablespoons (56.7 g)

Manuka	45 drops
Chamomile (Roman)	15 drops
Cornstarch	4 tablespoons (56.7 g)

Champaca Flower	35 drops
Manuka	25 drops
Cornstarch	4 tablespoons (56.7 g)

Champaca Flower	30 drops
Manuka	20 drops
Cabreuva	10 drops
Cornstarch	4 tablespoons (56.7 g)

Champaca Flower	30 drops
Manuka	20 drops
Spikenard	10 drops
Cornstarch	4 tablespoons (56.7 g)

Manuka	20 drops
Rosewood	20 drops
Champaca Flower	20 drops
Cornstarch	4 tablespoons (56.7 g)

FRESHEN-UP UNDERARM DEODORANTS

To help keep you smelling great all day, try one of these deodorants. First, apply five drops of aloe vera juice to each underarm, then combine the formula and rub in well. Each formula is for one underarm. Finish by dabbing on some cornstarch or arrowroot powder to dry off any remaining oil.

After a woman shaves her underarms, it is advisable to wait at least fifteen minutes before applying the deodorant to avoid any burning sensation.

| Manuka | 2 drops |
| Vanilla (CO_2) | 1 drop |

| Manuka | 2 drops |
| Rosewood | 1 drop |

Manuka	1 drop
Neroli	1 drop
Helichrysum	1 drop

| Champaca Flower | 2 drops |
| Manuka | 1 drop |

| Chamomile (Roman) | 1 drop |
| Manuka | 1 drop |

Lavender	1 drop
Neroli	1 drop
Manuka	1 drop

FRESHEN-UP UNDERARM DEODORANTS ROLL-ON

Choose one of these formulas. Place the essential oils into a small glass roll-on bottle. Apply five drops of aloe vera juice to each underarm, then roll on the deodorant. To dry any remaining oil, rub in well a small amount of cornstarch or arrowroot powder.

After a woman shaves her underarms, it is advisable to wait at least fifteen minutes before applying the deodorant to avoid any burning sensation. Place a label on the roll-on bottle and store in a dark, cool place.

| Manuka | 70 drops |
| Rosewood | 30 drops |

| Manuka | 80 drops |
| Vanilla (CO_2) | 20 drops |

| Manuka | 80 drops |
| Champaca Flower | 20 drops |

Manuka	70 drops
Helichrysum	20 drops
Rosewood	10 drops

Manuka	70 drops
Spikenard	15 drops
Vanilla (CO_2)	15 drops

| Manuka | 80 drops |
| Neroli | 20 drops |

HAIR RINSE

To bring out the shine in your hair, rinse with one of these hair formulas. Mix all the ingredients together and shake well before using. Apply a small portion to the scalp and hair after shampooing. Leave on for the duration of the shower, then rinse off. Notice the difference with each washing. Place a label on the bottle and store the remaining hair rinse in a dark, cool place.

Manuka	5 drops
Spearmint	5 drops
Cedarwood (Atlas)	4 drops
Lavender	3 drops
Tangerine	3 drops
Aloe Vera Juice	1 tablespoon (15 ml)
Apple Cider Vinegar	1 tablespoon (15 ml)
Water	28 ounces (840 ml)

Sage (Spanish)	5 drops
Spruce	5 drops
Spearmint	5 drops
Copaiba	5 drops
Aloe Vera Juice	1 tablespoon (15 ml)
Apple Cider Vinegar	1 tablespoon (15 ml)
Water	28 ounces (840 ml)

Litsea Cubeba	8 drops
Patchouli	7 drops
Chamomile (Roman)	5 drops
Aloe Vera Juice	1 tablespoon (15 ml)
Apple Cider Vinegar	1 tablespoon (15 ml)
Water	28 ounces (840 ml)

Copaiba	8 drops
Cedarwood (Atlas)	5 drops
Spearmint	5 drops
Juniper Berry	2 drops
Aloe Vera Juice	1 tablespoon (15 ml)
Apple Cider Vinegar	1 tablespoon (15 ml)
Water	28 ounces (840 ml)

Rosemary	5 drops
Chamomile (Roman)	5 drops
Lavender	5 drops
Palmarosa	5 drops
Aloe Vera Juice	1 tablespoon (15 ml)
Apple Cider Vinegar	1 tablespoon (15 ml)
Water	28 ounces (840 ml)

Helichrysum	6 drops
Spearmint	5 drops
Spruce	5 drops
Cedarwood (Atlas)	4 drops
Aloe Vera Juice	1 tablespoon (15 ml)
Apple Cider Vinegar	1 tablespoon (15 ml)
Water	28 ounces (840 ml)

MATTRESS REFRESHERS

A mattress can harbor many undesirable organisms like dust mites, lice, bed bugs, and all types of bacteria. These powders are helpful to freshen and sanitize the mattress.

Choose one of these formulas. Measure $1/2$ cup (4 ounces or 113.4 grams) of bicarbonate of soda and add the essential oils. Mix well and pour into a jar or container. Tighten the cap and let the formula sit for a day, so the scent of the oils can permeate the powder.

Sprinkle the powder on the mattress. Determine the amount to use by your preference for a lighter or stronger scent. Allow the powder to remain on the mattress for at least a few hours. Afterward, you can remove the powder with a vacuum cleaner. Place a label on the jar and store any remaining powder in a dark, cool place.

Lavender	20 drops
Marjoram	20 drops
Cedarwood (Atlas)	20 drops
Bicarbonate of Soda	$^1/_2$ cup (113.4 g)

Spruce	20 drops
Litsea Cubeba	15 drops
Amyris	15 drops
Clove Bud	10 drops
Bicarbonate of Soda	$^1/_2$ cup (113.4 g)

Lavender	40 drops
Eucalyptus Citriodora	10 drops
Cinnamon Leaf	5 drops
Spearmint	5 drops
Bicarbonate of Soda	$^1/_2$ cup (113.4 g)

Mandarin	20 drops
Lemon	20 drops
Lavender	10 drops
Cedarwood (Atlas)	10 drops
Bicarbonate of Soda	$^1/_2$ cup (113.4 g)

Fir Needles	25 drops
Spruce	25 drops
Clove Bud	5 drops
Cedarwood (Atlas)	5 drops
Bicarbonate of Soda	$^1/_2$ cup (113.4 g)

Eucalyptus Citriodora	20 drops
Tangerine	15 drops
Cedarwood (Atlas)	15 drops
Clove Bud	10 drops
Bicarbonate of Soda	$^1/_2$ cup (113.4 g)

Lemon	20 drops
Grapefruit	20 drops
Cedarwood (Atlas)	10 drops
Clove Bud	5 drops
Spearmint	5 drops
Bicarbonate of Soda	$^1/_2$ cup (113.4 g)

Lavender	40 drops
Spearmint	10 drops
Cedarwood (Atlas)	10 drops
Bicarbonate of Soda	$^1/_2$ cup (113.4 g)

Litsea Cubeba	20 drops
Eucalyptus Citriodora	15 drops
Tangerine	10 drops
Grapefruit	8 drops
Patchouli	7 drops
Bicarbonate of Soda	$^1/_2$ cup (113.4 g)

Lemon	20 drops
Tangerine	15 drops
Clove Bud	15 drops
Cedarwood (Atlas)	10 drops
Bicarbonate of Soda	$^1/_2$ cup (113.4 g)

MOSQUITO-BANDITO RELIEF

After you've been bitten by a mosquito, apply a few drops of aloe vera juice on the area, then select one of these formulas and rub it into the skin.

Rosewood	1 drop
Palmarosa	1 drop
Helichrysum	1 drop

Rosewood	1 drop
Lemon	1 drop
Marjoram	1 drop

Amyris	1 drop
Rosewood	1 drop
Helichrysum	1 drop

Amyris	1 drop
Palmarosa	1 drop
Marjoram	1 drop

Cumin	1 drop
Rosewood	1 drop
Marjoram	1 drop

Rosewood	1 drop
Guaiacwood	1 drop
Marjoram	1 drop

Marjoram	1 drop
Amyris	1 drop
Helichrysum	1 drop

Marjoram	1 drop
Rosewood	1 drop
Helichrysum	1 drop

Cumin	1 drop
Frankincense	1 drop
Helichrysum	1 drop

Cumin	1 drop
Marjoram	1 drop
Palmarosa	1 drop

PRE-ELECTRIC SHAVING POWDERS

Choose one of these formulas. Pour 1/2 cup (4 ounces or 113.4 grams) of cornstarch into a wide-mouthed glass jar. Stir the essential oils in well, cap the jar, and let the formula sit for several hours before using. Apply the powder to the area before shaving. Place a label on the jar and store the remaining powder in a dark, cool place.

Spruce	30 drops
Myrtle	30 drops
Rosewood	30 drops
Cornstarch	1/2 cup (113.4 g)

Mandarin	40 drops
Rosewood	30 drops
Neroli	20 drops
Cornstarch	1/2 cup (113.4 g)

Cypress	40 drops
Litsea Cubeba	40 drops
Patchouli	10 drops
Cornstarch	1/2 cup (113.4 g)

Spruce	40 drops
Rosewood	40 drops
Pine	10 drops
Cornstarch	1/2 cup (113.4 g)

Peppermint	40 drops
Eucalyptus Radiata	35 drops
Mandarin	15 drops
Cornstarch	1/2 cup (113.4 g)

Rosewood	30 drops
Lemon	25 drops
Mandarin	25 drops
Cedarwood (Atlas)	10 drops
Cornstarch	1/2 cup (113.4 g)

Spruce	30 drops
Eucalyptus Radiata	30 drops
Amyris	30 drops
Cornstarch	1/2 cup (113.4 g)

Mandarin	40 drops
Litsea Cubeba	30 drops
Pine	10 drops
Patchouli	10 drops
Cornstarch	1/2 cup (113.4 g)

Lavender	30 drops
Spearmint	30 drops
Basil (Sweet)	30 drops
Cornstarch	$1/2$ cup (113.4 g)

Spearmint	35 drops
Dill	20 drops
Mandarin	20 drops
Neroli	15 drops
Cornstarch	$1/2$ cup (113.4 g)

Geranium	30 drops
Rosewood	30 drops
Mandarin	30 drops
Cornstarch	$1/2$ cup (113.4 g)

Lemon	25 drops
Peppermint	25 drops
Rosewood	25 drops
Dill	15 drops
Cornstarch	$1/2$ cup (113.4 g)

SHAVING CREAMS

Choose one of these creams. To prepare, place the shea butter into a small wide-mouthed glass jar. Put the jar in a small pot of water, and warm on a low temperature. When the butter is melted, add the carrier oil, mix well, and remove from the heat. As the mixture cools, add the essential oils, stir well, and cap the jar. Apply a small amount to the skin, rub in, and shave. Place a label on the jar and store the remaining cream in a dark, cool place.

Sandalwood	10 drops
Litsea Cubeba	10 drops
Shea Butter	2 tablespoons (30 ml)
Carrier Oil	3 tablespoons (45 ml)

Fir Needles	5 drops
Spearmint	5 drops
Cedarwood (Atlas)	5 drops
Pine	5 drops
Shea Butter	2 tablespoons (30 ml)
Carrier Oil	3 tablespoons (45 ml)

Rosewood	7 drops
Litsea Cubeba	7 drops
Patchouli	6 drops
Shea Butter	2 tablespoons (30 ml)
Carrier Oil	3 tablespoons (45 ml)

Rosewood	10 drops
Lavender	10 drops
Shea Butter	2 tablespoons (30 ml)
Carrier Oil	3 tablespoons (45 ml)

Copaiba	10 drops
Peppermint	10 drops
Shea Butter	2 tablespoons (30 ml)
Carrier Oil	3 tablespoons (45 ml)

Spruce	13 drops
Coriander	7 drops
Shea Butter	2 tablespoons (30 ml)
Carrier Oil	3 tablespoons (45 ml)

Rosewood	5 drops
Palmarosa	5 drops
Cedarwood (Atlas)	5 drops
Spearmint	5 drops
Shea Butter	2 tablespoons (30 ml)
Carrier Oil	3 tablespoons (45 ml)

Spruce	6 drops
Pine	5 drops
Cedarwood (Atlas)	5 drops
Orange	4 drops
Shea Butter	2 tablespoons (30 ml)
Carrier Oil	3 tablespoons (45 ml)

Peppermint	7 drops
Eucalyptus Radiata	7 drops
Spruce	3 drops
Lavender	3 drops
Shea Butter	2 tablespoons (30 ml)
Carrier Oil	3 tablespoons (45 ml)

Fir Needles	6 drops
Spearmint	6 drops
Patchouli	4 drops
Litsea Cubeba	4 drops
Shea Butter	2 tablespoons (30 ml)
Carrier Oil	3 tablespoons (45 ml)

Grapefruit	7 drops
Neroli	7 drops
Rosewood	6 drops
Shea Butter	2 tablespoons (30 ml)
Carrier Oil	3 tablespoons (45 ml)

Spruce	9 drops
Fir Needles	7 drops
Pine	4 drops
Shea Butter	2 tablespoons (30 ml)
Carrier Oil	3 tablespoons (45 ml)

Geranium	7 drops
Rosewood	7 drops
Cedarwood (Atlas)	6 drops
Shea Butter	2 tablespoons (30 ml)
Carrier Oil	3 tablespoons (45 ml)

Peppermint	8 drops
Neroli	6 drops
Dill	6 drops
Shea Butter	2 tablespoons (30 ml)
Carrier Oil	3 tablespoons (45 ml)

TOOTH POWDERS

Make your own natural tooth powder that you can flavor according to your taste preference.

Choose one of these formulas. Measure 4 tablespoons (2 ounces or 56.7 grams) of arrowroot powder, pour into a small wide-mouthed glass jar, add the essential oils, and stir well. Then tighten the cap, and let the powder sit for a day. Mix again before using, and brush your teeth with a small amount each time. Place a label on the jar and store in a dark, cool place.

Helichrysum	20 drops
Arrowroot Powder	4 tablespoons (56.7 g)

Spearmint	15 drops
Sage (Spanish)	5 drops
Arrowroot Powder	4 tablespoons (56.7 g)

Fennel (Sweet)	8 drops
Spearmint	8 drops
Cinnamon Leaf	4 drops
Arrowroot Powder	4 tablespoons (56.7 g)

Spearmint	15 drops
Cinnamon Leaf	5 drops
Arrowroot Powder	4 tablespoons (56.7 g)

Helichrysum	10 drops
Peppermint	10 drops
Arrowroot Powder	4 tablespoons (56.7 g)

Peppermint	15 drops
Rosemary	5 drops
Arrowroot Powder	4 tablespoons (56.7 g)

CHAPTER 9

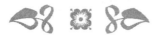

Carrier Oil Profiles

In aromatherapy, carrier oils play a key role by diluting the essential oils for use in massage, skin, and hair care preparations. These oils are beneficial in protecting the skin by moisturizing, soothing, softening, and nourishing the skin cells as the oil is absorbed deep into the skin layers. Whenever essential oils are applied topically, carrier oils must be combined with them to form a blend.

ALMOND (SWEET)

Botanical Name: *Prunus amygdalus, Prunus dulcis*

Family: *Rosaceae*

The oil is obtained from the nuts.

Plant Description: Sweet almond is a medium-size tree that grows to a height of about 35 feet (10.5 meters) and has pinkish-white flowers, followed by green fruits, each containing a nut. There are approximately fifty species of wild almond trees, but only a few varieties produce a sweet kernel.

Practical Uses

Skin and hair care; moisturizing to the skin

APRICOT KERNEL

Botanical Name: *Armeniaca vulgaris, Prunus armeniaca*

Family: *Rosaceae*

The oil is obtained from the kernels.

Plant Description: The apricot tree grows to a height of about 35 feet (10.5 meters) and has white to pink flowers that develop into orange-yellow fruit, with a kernel inside.

Practical Uses

Skin and hair care; moisturizing to the skin

AVOCADO

Botanical Name: *Persea americana, Persea gratissima*

Family: *Lauraceae*

The oil is obtained from the kernels.

Plant Description: Avocado is an evergreen tree that grows to a height of about 30 to 60 feet (9 to 18 meters), has dark-green oval, leathery leaves and greenish-yellow flowers that develop into yellow, green, red, or purple fruit. The pulp is soft and buttery with a large kernel inside.

Practical Uses

Skin and hair care; moisturizing; removes impurities from the skin

Comments

For massage blends, it is best to mix approximately 20 percent of avocado oil with another carrier oil. For skin and hair care purposes, avocado oil can be applied without being diluted.

EVENING PRIMROSE

Botanical Name: *Oenothera biennis*

Family: *Onagraceae*

The oil and CO_2 extract are obtained from the seeds.

Plant Description: Evening primrose is a plant that grows to a height of about 1 to 8 feet (0.3 to 2.4 meters), has long, pointed leaves and many fragrant yellow flowers that open at dusk to attract night-flying insects for pollination. Following the flowers are capsules containing many small brownish-colored seeds.

Practical Uses

Helps reduce premenstrual stress; relieves menstrual pain; reduces inflammation; skin and hair care; moisturizing and soothing to the skin

Comments

For massage blends, it is best to mix approximately 20 percent of evening primrose with another carrier oil. For skin and hair purposes, evening primrose oil can be applied without being diluted.

HAZELNUT

Botanical Name: *Corylus avellana*

Family: *Betulaceae*

The oil and CO_2 extract are obtained from the nuts.

Plant Description: Hazelnut is a tree that grows to a height of about 12 to 30 feet (3.6 to 9 meters), has green leaves, light-yellow catkins, and red female flowers that develop into nuts. Hazelnut is also known as filbert nut and cob nut.

Practical Uses

Skin and hair care; moisturizes, softens, repairs dry and damaged skin

JOJOBA

Botanical Name: *Simmondsia chinensis*

Family: *Buxaceae*

The vegetable wax/oil is obtained from the beans.

Plant Description: Jojoba is an evergreen shrub that grows to a height of about 3 to 18 feet (0.9 to 5.4 meters) and has small leathery leaves. There are male and female plants. The male flowers are yellow; the female flowers are green and develop into olive-shaped, dark-brown, nutlike fruits containing seeds. The seeds are called goat nuts. Jojoba plants can live up to 200 years.

Practical Uses

Skin care; moisturizes and softens dry skin; helps to reduce stretch marks; suntanning oil for those who burn easily; scalp and hair care

Comments

For massage blends, it is best to mix approximately 50 percent of jojoba oil with another carrier oil. For skin and hair care purposes, jojoba oil can be applied without being diluted.

MACADAMIA NUT

Botanical Name: *Macadamia integrifolia, Macadamia ternifolia, Macadamia tetraphylla*

Family: *Proteaceae*

The oil is obtained from the nuts.

Plant Description: Macadamia is an evergreen tree. *Macadamia integrifolia* grows to about 60 feet (18 meters) and has glossy, oblong leaves. *Macadamia ternifolia* grows to a height of about 15 feet (4.5 meters) and has dark-green glossy leaves. *Macadamia tetraphylla* reaches 40 to 50 feet (12 to 15 meters) and has dark-green leaves. Depending on the variety, the trees have clusters of white, pink, or pale brown flowers that produce hard-shelled brown nuts. The nuts are also known as Queensland nut, Australian nut, bauple nut, and bopple nut.

Practical Uses

Skin and hair care; softens and restores the skin

SESAME

Botanical Name: *Sesamum indicum, Sesamum orientale*

Family: *Pedaliaceae*

The oil is obtained from the seeds.

Plant Description: Sesame is a plant that grows to a height of about 3 to 6 feet (.09 to 1.8 meters) and has white or pink tubular flowers with purple spots. The color of the seeds can be white, yellow, red, brown, or black. There are thirty-seven species of the plant. Sesame is also referred to as sim-sim. Sesame oil is also known as benne oil, gingle oil, and teel oil.

Practical Uses

Skin care; moisturizing and soothing to the skin; scalp and hair care

CHAPTER 10

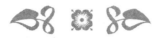

Essential Oil Profiles

ALLSPICE BERRY

Botanical Name: *Pimenta dioica, Pimenta officinalis*

Family: *Myrtaceae*

The essential oil is obtained from the dried unripe berries.

Plant Description: Allspice is an evergreen tree that grows to a height of about 30 to 70 feet (9 to 21 meters) and has leathery leaves with small white flowers that develop into aromatic berries that turn dark brown when ripe.

Aromatherapy Uses

Warming, improves circulation; calms the nerves, removes stress; promotes a restful sleep; vapors open the sinus and breathing passages; mood uplifting; improves mental clarity and the memory; improves digestion; purifying, helps in the reduction of cellulite; loosens tight muscles; lessens pain

Comments

Allspice berry oil is milder to the skin than the leaf oil.

Precaution

People with dry or sensitive skin may require additional carrier oil when applying allspice berry essential oil topically.

AMYRIS

Botanical Name: *Amyris balsamifera*

Family: *Rutaceae*

The essential oil is obtained from the wood chips.

Plant Description: Amyris is an evergreen tree that grows to a height of about 60 feet (18 meters) and has clusters of white flowers that develop into an edible, bluish-black fruit.

Aromatherapy Uses

Cooling; calming; reduces anxiety, stress, and tension; promotes a peaceful state; helps to deepen the breathing; reviving; improves mental clarity; loosens tight muscles; used as a fixative to hold the scent of a fragrance

ANISE

Botanical Name: *Anisum officinalis, Anisum officinarum, Pimpinella anisum*

Family: *Apiaceae*

The essential oil is obtained from the seeds.

Plant Description: The anise plant reaches a height of about 2 feet (0.6 meter) and has small white flowers, followed by seeds.

Aromatherapy Uses

Calming, relaxing; promotes a restful sleep; vapors help open the sinus and breathing passages; mood uplifting; improves digestion, soothes the intestines, relieves flatulence and aerophagy (excessive swallowing of air); lessens pain and helps relieve menstrual discomfort; increases lactation

Precaution

People with dry or sensitive skin may require additional carrier oil when applying the essential oil topically. Anise tends to slow down the reflexes. Avoid driving or doing anything that requires full attention after using the oil. Use small amounts.

BASIL (SWEET)

Botanical Name: *Ocimum basilicum*

Family: *Lamiaceae*

The essential oil is obtained from the whole plant.

The CO_2 extract is obtained from the leaves.

Plant Description: Sweet basil is a bushy plant that grows to a height of about 2 feet (0.6 meter) and has white, blue, or purple flowers.

Aromatherapy Uses

Cooling; calming, reduces stress; promotes a restful sleep, encourages dreaming; helpful for meditation; mood uplifting; improves mental clarity and the memory, sharpens the senses; improves digestion; purifying, helps in the reduction of cellulite; lessens pain; increases lactation; neutralizes toxins from insect bites, soothes insect bites

Precaution

People with dry or sensitive skin may require additional carrier oil when applying basil essential oil topically. Use small amounts.

BERGAMOT

Botanical Name: *Citrus bergamia*

Family: *Rutaceae*

The essential oil is obtained from the peel of the fruit.

Plant Description: Bergamot is an evergreen citrus tree that grows to a height of about 15 feet (4.5 meters) and bears nonedible green to yellow fruit.

Aromatherapy Uses

Cooling; balancing; calming; relieves anxiety, nervous tension, and stress; promotes a restful sleep; mood uplifting, refreshing; helps to relieve fatigue; improves mental clarity, alertness, sharpens the senses; purifying, helps in the reduction of cellulite

Precaution

People with dry or sensitive skin may require additional carrier oil when using the essential oil topically. Bergamot is phototoxic. Avoid exposure to direct sunlight for several hours after applying the oil on the skin.

BLACK PEPPER

Botanical Name: *Piper nigrum*

Family: *Piperaceae*

The essential oil and CO_2 extract are obtained from the berries.

Plant Description: Black pepper is a tropical climbing vine that grows to a height of about 10 feet (3 meters) and has clusters of small white flowers. As the berries ripen, they turn from green to orange to red. After the berries are picked, they are left in the sun to dry, which turns their color to black.

Aromatherapy Uses

Warming, increases circulation; reviving, stimulating, improves mental clarity; improves digestion in small amounts; loosens tight muscles; improves the benefits of other oils that are used together with black pepper

Precaution

People with dry or sensitive skin may require additional carrier oil when applying black pepper essential oil topically. Use small amounts.

CABREUVA

Botanical Name: *Myrocarpus fastigiatus*

Family: *Fabaceae*

The essential oil is obtained from the wood chips.

Plant Description: Cabreuva is a tropical tree that grows to a height of about 50 feet (15 meters).

Aromatherapy Uses

Warming; calming, reduces stress and tension; helps to breathe easier; mood uplifting, euphoric, aphrodisiac, reviving; improves mental clarity and alertness; loosens tight muscles, reduces pain

CAJEPUT

Botanical Name: *Melaleuca cajuputi, Melaleuca leucadendron, Melaleuca minor*

Family: *Myrtaceae*

The essential oil is obtained from the leaves and buds.

Plant Description: Cajeput is an evergreen tree that grows to a height of about 50 to 100 feet (15 to 30 meters), has a papery bark and narrow leaves.

Aromatherapy Uses

Slightly warming, improves circulation; calming, reduces stress; promotes a restful sleep; vapors open the sinus and breathing passages; deepens the breathing; relieves aches and pains; repels insects

CARDAMOM

Botanical Name: *Elettaria cardamomum*

Family: *Zingiberaceae*

The essential oil and CO_2 extract are obtained from the seeds.

Plant Description: Cardamom is a plant that grows to a height of about 10 feet (3 meters) and has small yellow flowers.

Aromatherapy Uses

Warming, improves circulation; mood uplifting; energizing, improves mental clarity and the memory; improves physical strength, increases sexual strength; improves digestion, soothes the intestines, relieves flatulence; relieves pain, menstrual pains, and cramps

CEDARWOOD (ATLAS)

Botanical Name: *Cedrus atlantica*

Family: *Pinaceae*

The essential oil is obtained from the wood.

Plant Description: Cedarwood is an evergreen tree that grows to a height of about 130 to 140 feet (39 to 42 meters), has bluish-green needle-like leaves and light green cones that mature to a brownish-gray color.

Aromatherapy Uses

Cooling; calming, relieves anxiety and nervous tension; promotes a restful sleep, encourages dreaming; helpful for meditation; helps to breathe easier, opens the sinus and breathing passages, eases chest congestion when rubbed on the chest; improves mental clarity; loosens tight

muscles, lessens pain; repels insects; used as a fixative to hold the scent of a fragrance

CELERY

Botanical Name: *Apium graveolens*

Family: *Apiaceae*

The essential oil and CO_2 extract are obtained from the seeds.

Plant Description: Celery is a biennial plant that grows to a height of about 1 to 2 feet (0.3 to 0.6 meters) and has green-white flowers that develop into seeds.

Aromatherapy Uses

Cooling; calming, relaxing; promotes a restful sleep; purifying, helps in the reduction of cellulite

Precaution

Celery tends to slow down the reflexes. Avoid driving or doing anything that requires full attention after using the essential oil. Due to celery's detoxifying effect, use in small amounts.

CHAMOMILE (ROMAN)

Botanical Name: *Anthemis nobilis, Chamaemelum nobile*

Family: *Asteraceae*

The essential oil is obtained from the flowers and leaves.

Plant Description: The Roman chamomile plant grows to a height of about 1 foot (0.3 meter), has feathery leaves and white flowers with a yellow disk in the center, similar in appearance to daisies.

Aromatherapy Uses

Calming; promotes a restful sleep; mood uplifting; improves digestion, soothes the intestines; lessens pain, relieves menstrual discomfort, soothes inflammation; healing to the skin; soothes insect bites

CHAMPACA FLOWER

Botanical Name: *Michelia alba, Michelia champaca*

Family: *Magnoliaceae*

The essential oil is obtained from the flowers.

Plant Description: Champaca is an evergreen tree that grows to a height of about 65 feet (19.5 meters), has long, glossy leaves and small, fragrant white, yellow, or orange flowers that develop into fruit.

Aromatherapy Uses

Warming; calming, reduces stress, promotes a peaceful state; helps to breathe easier; mood uplifting, euphoric; used as a fixative to hold the scent of a fragrance

CINNAMON LEAF

Botanical Name: *Cinnamomum verum, Cinnamomum zeylanicum*

Family: *Lauraceae*

The essential oil is obtained from the leaves.

Plant Description: Cinnamon is a tropical ever-

green tree that grows to a height of about 25 to 60 feet (7.5 to 18 meters), has shiny green leathery leaves and clusters of small yellow flowers that develop into light blue berries.

Aromatherapy Uses

Warming, improves circulation; calming, relaxing, reduces stress; mood uplifting, reviving, helps to relieve a fatigued state; improves digestion; purifying, helps in the reduction of cellulite; loosens tight muscles, lessens pain; repels insects

Precaution

People with dry or sensitive skin may require additional carrier oil when applying cinnamon leaf essential oil topically. Use small amounts.

CITRONELLA

Botanical Name: *Andropogon nardus, Cymbopogon nardus*

Family: *Poaceae*

The essential oil is obtained from the grass.

Plant Description: Citronella is an aromatic tall grass.

Aromatherapy Uses

Cooling; calming, reduces stress; mood uplifting; mental stimulant, improves mental clarity and alertness; repels insects

Precaution

People with dry or sensitive skin may require additional carrier oil when using the essential oil topically. Citronella is phototoxic. Avoid exposure to direct sunlight for several hours after applying the oil on the skin.

CLARY SAGE

Botanical Name: *Salvia sclarea*

Family: *Lamiaceae*

The essential oil is obtained from the flowering tops.

Plant Description: Clary sage is a plant that grows to a height of about 3 feet (0.9 meter) and has whorls of pink, white, or blue flowers, depending on the variety.

Aromatherapy Uses

Calming, relieves stress and tension; promotes a restful sleep; mood uplifting, aphrodisiac; increases sexual strength; improves digestion; relieves menstrual pain and cramps, regulates the female reproductive system

Precaution

Due to the relaxing effect of the essential oil, clary sage should not be used before driving or doing anything that requires full attention. Clary sage can dull the senses. Use small amounts.

CLOVE BUD

Botanical Name: *Eugenia aromatica, Eugenia caryophyllata, Eugenia caryophyllus, Syzygium aromaticum*

Family: *Myrtaceae*

The essential oil and CO_2 extract are obtained from the buds.

Plant Description: Clove is a tropical evergreen tree that grows to a height of about 40 to 70 feet (12 to 21 meters), has aromatic, dark-green leathery leaves and bright pink buds that bloom into yellow flowers, followed by purple berries.

Aromatherapy Uses

Heating; vapors open the sinus and breathing passages; mood uplifting, aphrodisiac, reviving; mental stimulant, improves mental clarity and the memory; improves digestion, relieves flatulence; reduces pain by numbing the area; repels insects

Comments

The oil from clove bud is more suitable for use in aromatherapy, since it is less irritating than the leaf and stem oils.

Precaution

People with dry or sensitive skin may require additional carrier oil when applying clove bud essential oil topically. Use small amounts.

COPAIBA

Botanical Name: *Copaifera officinalis*

Family: *Fabaceae*

The resin and essential oil are obtained from the tree trunk.

Plant Description: Copaiba is a tropical evergreen tree that grows to a height of about 60 to 100 feet (18 to 30 meters) and has small yellow flowers, followed by fruit that turn from brown to red.

Aromatherapy Uses

Warming, improves circulation; calming, reduces stress, promotes a peaceful state of mind and a restful sleep; helpful for meditation; opens the breathing passages for deeper breathing; mood uplifting; improves mental clarity and alertness; soothes the intestines; healing and moisturizing to the skin; used as a fixative to hold the scent of a fragrance

CUMIN

Botanical Name: *Cuminum cyminum, Cuminum odorum*

Family: *Apiaceae*

The essential oil is obtained from the seeds and fruit.

The CO_2 extract is obtained from the seeds.

Plant Description: Cumin is a plant that grows to a height of about 1 foot (0.3 meter), has threadlike leaves and small white or pink flowers, followed by aromatic seeds.

Aromatherapy Uses

Warming, improves circulation, calming, reduces stress; helpful for meditation; mood uplifting, euphoric; reviving, helps to relieve fatigue; improves digestion, relieves flatulence; purifying, helps in the reduction of cellulite; relieves pain; soothes insect bites

Precaution

People with dry or sensitive skin may require additional carrier oil when using the essential oil topically. Use small amounts. Cumin is phototoxic. Avoid exposure to direct sunlight for several hours after applying the oil on the skin.

CYPRESS

Botanical Name: *Cupressus sempervirens*

Family: *Cupressaceae*

The essential oil is obtained from the leaves and twigs.

Plant Description: Cypress is an evergreen tree that grows to a height of about 80 to 160 feet (24 to 48 meters), has dark-green leaves and cones that turn brown when mature.

Aromatherapy Uses

Balancing to the nervous system; calming, relieves nervous tension and stress; promotes a restful sleep; helps the breathing; mood uplifting, refreshing; improves mental clarity and alertness; purifying, helps in the reduction of cellulite; contracts weak connective tissue; relieves muscle tension; regulates the female reproductive and hormonal systems; lessens perspiration

DILL

Botanical Name: *Anethum graveolens, Fructus anethi, Peucedanum graveolens*

Family: *Apiaceae*

Dill seed essential oil and CO_2 extract are obtained from the seeds.

Dill weed essential oil is obtained from the whole plant.

Plant Description: Dill is a plant that grows to a height of about 3 feet (0.9 meter) and has small yellow flowers.

Aromatherapy Uses

Calming, relaxing; promotes a restful sleep; improves digestion, soothes and freshens the intestines, relieves flatulence and fermentation; relieves pain and menstrual discomfort; increases lactation; repels insects

Precaution

Dill tends to slow down the reflexes. Avoid driving or doing anything that requires full attention after using the essential oil.

EUCALYPTUS CITRIODORA

Botanical Name: *Eucalyptus citriodora*

Family: *Myrtaceae*

The essential oil is obtained from the leaves and twigs.

Plant Description: *Eucalyptus citriodora* is an evergreen tree that grows to a height of about 90 to 120 feet (27 to 36 meters) and has a smooth white bark, narrow pointed leaves with a lemony scent, and white flowers.

Aromatherapy Uses

Calming; mood uplifting, reviving, helps to relieve a fatigued state

EUCALYPTUS RADIATA

Botanical Name: *Eucalyptus radiata*

Family: *Myrtaceae*

The essential oil is obtained from the leaves and twigs.

Plant Description: *Eucalyptus radiata* is a tree that grows to a height of about 150 to 170 feet (45 to 51 meters), has a dark bark, narrow green aromatic leaves, and cream-colored flowers.

Aromatherapy Uses

Cooling; stimulating to the nervous system; vapors open the sinus and breathing passages, deepens the breathing; improves circulation; refreshing, reviving, energizing, improves mental clarity and alertness; relieves pain, aching, and sore muscles; repels insects

Comments

Eucalyptus radiata is considered to be gentler than the common variety of *Eucalyptus globulus*.

FENNEL (SWEET)

Botanical Name: *Anethum foeniculum, Foeniculum officinale, Foeniculum vulgare*

Family: *Apiaceae*

The essential oil and CO_2 extract are obtained from the seeds.

Plant Description: Fennel is an aromatic plant that grows to a height of about 3 to 7 feet (0.9 to 2.1 meters), has green feathery leaves and clusters of small yellow flowers that develop into brownish-gray seeds.

Aromatherapy Uses

Warming, improves circulation; reduces stress; promotes a restful sleep; helpful for breathing; improves the digestion, soothes and purifies the intestines, relieves flatulence and aerophagy (excessive swallowing of air); purifying, helps in the reduction of cellulite; relieves pain and menstrual discomfort; increases lactation; repels insects

Precaution

People with dry or sensitive skin may require additional carrier oil when applying the essential oil topically. Fennel tends to slow down the reflexes. Avoid driving or doing anything that requires full attention after using the oil. Use small amounts. Fennel should be avoided by people prone to epileptic seizures.

FIR NEEDLES

Botanical Name: *Abies alba* (*Silver fir*), *Abies balsamea* (*Fir balsam needles*), *Abies grandis* (*Grand fir*), *Pseudotsuga menziesii* (*Douglas fir*)

Family: *Pinaceae*

The essential oil is obtained from the needles.

Plant Description: Fir is an evergreen tree that grows to a height of about 100 to 300 feet (30 to 90 meters), has needlelike leaves, brown cones, and soft, odorless wood.

Aromatherapy Uses

Calming; vapors open the sinus and breathing passages; deepens the breathing; mood uplifting, refreshing, reviving; improves mental clarity; encourages communication; purifying, removes lymphatic deposits from the body, helps in the reduction of cellulite; lessens pain

FRANKINCENSE

Botanical Name: *Boswellia carteri, Boswellia sacra, Boswellia thurifera*

Family: *Burseraceae*

The resin, essential oil, and CO_2 extract are obtained from the bark resin.

Plant Description: Frankincense is a small tree that grows to a height of about 20 feet (6 meters), has glossy leaves and white flowers.

Aromatherapy Uses

Calming, relaxing; promotes a restful sleep; helpful for meditation; vapors open the sinus and breathing passages; mood uplifting, brings out feelings; reduces inflammation; soothes and heals inflamed skin, bruises, and burns

GALBANUM

Botanical Name: *Ferula galbaniflua, Ferula gumosa, Ferula rubricaulis*

Family: *Apiaceae*

The resin and essential oil are obtained from the bark.

The CO_2 extract is obtained from the resin.

Plant Description: Galbanum is a plant that grows to a height of about 3 feet (0.9 meter), has long grayish-green hairy leaves and umbels of very small yellow flowers that bear seeds.

Aromatherapy Uses

Calming, reduces stress; mood uplifting; relieves pain and inflammation

GERANIUM

Botanical Name: *Pelargonium graveolens*

Family: *Geraniaceae*

The essential oil is obtained from the leaves, stems, and flowers.

Plant Description: Geranium is a small plant that grows to a height of about 3 feet (0.9 meter), has fragrant leaves and red, pink, and other colored flowers.

Aromatherapy Uses

Cooling; calming to the nervous system in small amounts, stimulating in large amounts; reduces tension; mood uplifting; encourages communication; stimulates the adrenal glands; purifying, helps in the reduction of cellulite; lessens pain and inflammation; soothes itchy skin; repels insects; soothes insect bites; kills lice and ticks

GINGER

Botanical Name: *Amomum zingiber, Zingiber officinale*

Family: *Zingiberaceae*

The essential oil and CO_2 extract are obtained from the roots.

Plant Description: Ginger is a plant that grows to a height of about 3 feet (.09 meter) and has white or yellow flowers.

Aromatherapy Uses

Warming, improves circulation; mood uplifting; general stimulant to the entire body; improves mental clarity and the memory; relieves dizzi-ness and nausea caused by traveling; improves digestion, soothes the intestines, relieves flatulence, cleanses the bowels; loosens tight muscles, relieves aches and pains

Precaution

People with dry or sensitive skin may require additional carrier oil when applying ginger essential oil topically. Use small amounts.

GRAPEFRUIT

Botanical Name: *Citrus paradisi*

Family: *Rutaceae*

The essential oil is obtained from the peel of the fruit.

Plant Description: Grapefruit is an evergreen citrus tree that grows to a height of about 30 to 50 feet (9 to 15 meters), has glossy green leaves and fragrant white flowers that develop into large, edible yellow fruit.

Aromatherapy Uses

Cooling; reduces stress; mood uplifting, refreshing, reviving; improves mental clarity, awareness, and the memory; sharpens the senses; increases physical strength and energy; purifying, helps in the reduction of cellulite; balances fluids in the body

Precautions

People with dry or sensitive skin may require additional carrier oil when using the essential oil topically. Use small amounts. Grapefruit is phototoxic. Avoid exposure to direct sunlight for several hours after applying the oil on the skin.

GUAIACWOOD

Botanical Name: *Bulnesia sarmienti, Guaiacum officinale*

Family: *Zygophyllaceae*

The resin/essential oil is obtained from the wood.

Plant Description: Guaiacwood is an evergreen tree that grows to a height of about 30 to 40 feet (9 to 12 meters), has leathery leaves and clusters of small deep blue or purple flowers.

Aromatherapy Uses

Calming and relaxing, reduces stress and tension; promotes a restful sleep; helpful for meditation; mood uplifting; improves mental clarity; purifying to the tissues; reduces inflammation, soothes swollen and injured skin tissue; loosens tight muscles; soothes insect bites

Precaution

Guaiacwood tends to slow down the reflexes. Avoid driving or doing anything that requires full attention after using the resin or essential oil.

HELICHRYSUM (EVERLASTING OR IMMORTELLE)

Botanical Name: *Helichrysum angustifolium, Helichrysum italicum*

Family: *Asteraceae*

The essential oil is obtained from the flowers.

Plant Description: Helichrysum is an evergreen plant that grows to a height of about 2 feet (0.6 meters), has silvery-green leaves and clusters of daisylike yellow flowers.

Aromatherapy Uses

Cooling; relaxing, reduces stress; vapors open the sinus and breathing passages; mood uplifting, euphoric, reviving, strengthening; improves mental clarity and alertness; increases muscle endurance; relieves aches, pains, and menstrual discomfort; soothes insect bites

HYSSOP DECUMBENS

Botanical Name: *Hyssopus officinalis var. decumbens*

Family: *Lamiaceae*

The essential oil is obtained from the leaves and flowering tops.

Plant Description: Hyssop is a semi-evergreen bushy plant that grows to a height of about 1 to 4 feet (0.3 to 1.2 meters), has aromatic leaves and spikes of white, pink, blue, or dark purple flowers.

Aromatherapy Uses

Relaxing; vapors open the sinus and breathing passages; deepens the breathing; mood uplifting, reviving; improves mental clarity and alertness

Comments

Hyssopus decumbens is gentler than the essential oil variety of *Hyssopus officinalis*.

Precaution

Use small amounts. The essential oil should be avoided by people who are prone to epileptic seizures.

JUNIPER BERRY

Botanical Name: *Juniperus communis*

Family: *Cupressaceae*

The essential oil and CO_2 extract are obtained from the ripe berries.

Plant Description: Juniper is an evergreen bush that grows to a height of about 2 to 6 feet (0.6 to 1.8 meters), sometimes reaching as high as 25 feet (7.5 meters). The male trees have yellow cones, and the female trees have bluish-green cones. The silvery-green leaves are needlelike. The green berries take three years to ripen to a bluish-black color.

Aromatherapy Uses

Relaxing, reduces stress; mood uplifting, refreshing, reviving; improves mental clarity and the memory; purifying, cleansing to the intestines and the tissues in the body, reduces fluid retention, helps in the reduction of cellulite; lessens pain, painful swellings, painful menstruation; repels insects

Precaution

Because of juniper berry's strong stimulating effect on the kidneys, use small amounts. Avoid use on a person who has weak kidneys.

LAVENDER

Botanical Name: *Lavandula angustifolia, Lavandula officinalis, Lavandula vera*

Family: *Lamiaceae*

The essential oil and CO_2 extract are obtained from the flowers.

Plant Description: Lavender is an aromatic evergreen plant that grows to a height of about 3 feet (0.9 meters) and has spikes of lilac-colored flowers.

Aromatherapy Uses

Calming, lessens stress and tension; promotes a restful sleep; vapors open the sinus and breathing passages; mood uplifting; strengthening to the nerves, balances mood swings; improves digestion, soothing to the intestines; purifying, helps in the reduction of cellulite, gently removes fluid retention; relaxes the muscles, lessens aches and pains; reduces inflammation; healing to the skin, bruises, cuts, wounds, burns, sunburns, scars, sores, insect bites, and injuries; repels insects, kills lice

LEMON

Botanical Name: *Citrus limon*

Family: *Rutaceae*

The essential oil is obtained from the peel of the fruit.

Plant Description: Lemon is an evergreen citrus tree that grows to a height of about 10 to 20 feet (3 to 6 meters) and has fragrant white flowers that develop into edible yellow fruit.

Aromatherapy Uses

Cooling; calming, relaxing, reduces stress; promotes a restful sleep; mood uplifting, refreshing, reviving; improves mental clarity, alertness, and the memory; sharpens the senses; purifying, cleanses the tissues, reduces cellulite; soothes insect bites

Precaution

People with dry or sensitive skin may require additional carrier oil when using the essential oil topically. Use small amounts. Lemon is photo-toxic. Avoid exposure to direct sunlight for several hours after applying the oil on the skin.

LEMON MYRTLE

Botanical Name: *Backhousia citriodora*

Family: *Myrtaceae*

The essential oil is obtained from the leaves and branches.

Plant Description: Lemon myrtle is a bushy evergreen rainforest tree that grows to a height of about 30 to 50 feet (9 to 15 meters), has fragrant lemon-scented leaves and profuse clusters of cream-colored flowers.

Aromatherapy Uses

Warming; calming, relaxes the nerves, reduces stress and tension; helpful for meditation; vapors help open the sinus and breathing passages; mood uplifting, euphoric; refreshing, improves mental clarity and alertness; improves digestion; loosens tight muscles, relieves pain

Precaution

People with dry or sensitive skin may require additional carrier oil when applying lemon myrtle essential oil topically. Use small amounts.

LEMONGRASS

Botanical Name: *Cymbopogon citratus, Cymbopogon flexuosus*

Family: *Poaceae*

The essential oil is obtained from the whole plant.

Plant Description: Lemongrass is a grass that grows to a height of about 2 feet (0.6 meters), has swordlike leaves and an aromatic rhizome.

Aromatherapy Uses

Balancing to the nervous system; calming, reduces stress; promotes a restful sleep; vapors help open the sinus and breathing passages; mood uplifting; reviving, improves alertness; improves digestion; reduces inflammation and swollen tissues; contracts weak connective tissue, tones the skin; increases lactation; repels insects

Precaution

People with dry or sensitive skin may require additional carrier oil when applying lemongrass essential oil topically. Use small amounts.

LIME

Botanical Name: *Citrus aurantiifolia, Citrus limetta*

Family: *Rutaceae*

The essential oil is obtained from the peel of the fruit.

Plant Description: Lime is an evergreen citrus tree that grows to a height of about 10 feet (3 meters) and has fragrant, small white flowers that develop into edible green fruit with an acid pulp.

Aromatherapy Uses

Cooling; strengthening to the nerves; helpful when there is weakness in the body; reduces stress; mood uplifting, refreshing, reviving; improves mental clarity and alertness, sharpens the senses; purifying, helps in the reduction of cellulite; soothes insect bites

Precaution

People with dry or sensitive skin may require additional carrier oil when using the essential oil topically. Use small amounts. Lime is phototoxic. Avoid exposure to direct sunlight for several hours after applying the oil on the skin.

LITSEA CUBEBA

Botanical Name: *Litsea citrata, Litsea cubeba*

Family: *Lauraceae*

The essential oil is obtained from the fruit.

Plant Description: Litsea cubeba is a tropical evergreen tree that grows to a height of about 30 to 40 feet (9 to 12 meters), has lemony-scented leaves and white or yellow flowers that develop into small red or black berries.

Aromatherapy Uses

Cooling; calming, reduces stress; promotes a restful sleep; mood uplifting, euphoric, reviving; improves mental clarity and alertness; improves digestion; relieves pain

Precaution

People with dry or sensitive skin may require additional carrier oil when applying litsea cubeba essential oil topically. Use small amounts.

MANDARIN

Botanical Name: *Citrus nobilis, Citrus reticulata*

Family: *Rutaceae*

The essential oil is obtained from the peel of the fruit.

Plant Description: Mandarin is an evergreen citrus tree that grows to a height of about 10 to 25 feet (3 to 7.5 meters), has glossy leaves and fragrant white flowers that develop into edible orange fruit.

Aromatherapy Uses

Cooling; calming; promotes a restful sleep, encourages dreaming; mood uplifting, improves mental clarity and alertness, sharpens the mind; relieves emotional tension and stress, calms angry and irritable children; purifying, helps in the reduction of cellulite

Precaution

People with dry or sensitive skin may require additional carrier oil when using the essential oil topically. Use small amounts. Mandarin is phototoxic. Avoid exposure to direct sunlight for several hours after applying the oil on the skin.

MANUKA (NEW ZEALAND TEA TREE)

Botanical Name: *Leptospermum scoparium*

Family: *Myrtaceae*

The essential oil is obtained from the leaves and branches.

Plant Description: Manuka is an evergreen shrub that grows to a height of about 6 to10 feet

(1.8 to 3 meters), has small leaves and white or occasionally pink or red flowers.

Aromatherapy Uses

Calming, reduces stress and tension; helps to breathe easier; mood uplifting, euphoric, aphrodisiac; improves mental clarity; loosens tight muscles, relieves aches and pains; deodorant; healing to the skin

MARJORAM (SPANISH OR SWEET)

Botanical Name: *Thymus mastichina* (Spanish marjoram); *Majorana hortensis, Origanum majorana* (Sweet marjoram)

Family: *Lamiaceae*

The essential oil is obtained from the flowering tops and leaves.

Plant Description: Spanish marjoram is a bushy plant that grows to a height of about 1 foot (0.3 meter), and has small white flowers. Sweet marjoram is a bushy plant that grows to a height of about 2 feet (0.6 meter), has light-grayish-green leaves and white or purple flowers.

Aromatherapy Uses

Warming, improves circulation, dilates the blood vessels; relaxing, calms nervous tension; promotes a restful sleep; vapors open the sinus and breathing passages, deepens the breathing, especially helpful during colds and nasal congestion; improves digestion; relaxes tense muscles, relieves aches, pains, painful menstruation, inflammation, and spasms; soothes insect bites

Precaution

Due to the relaxing effect of the essential oil, marjoram should not be used before driving or doing anything that requires full attention. In large amounts, marjoram can dull the senses. Use small amounts.

MYRTLE

Botanical Name: *Myrtus communis*

Family: *Myrtaceae*

The essential oil is obtained from the leaves, twigs, and flowering tops.

Plant Description: Myrtle is an evergreen shrub that grows to a height of about 10 to18 feet (3 to 5.4 meters), has scented dark-green leaves and small, fragrant white or pink flowers with many yellow stamens.

Aromatherapy Uses

Calming; helpful for meditation; vapors open the sinus and breathing passages; mood uplifting, refreshing; relieves pain

NEROLI

Botanical Name: *Citrus aurantium*

Family: *Rutaceae*

The essential oil is obtained from the blossoms.

Plant Description: Bitter orange is an evergreen citrus tree that grows to a height of about 20 to 30 feet (6 to 9 meters) and has fragrant white flowers that yield neroli oil.

Aromatherapy Uses

Calms nervous tension, relaxes hyperactive children; promotes a restful sleep; mood uplifting, boosts confidence, helps soothe emotional upsets; soothes the intestines; helps to relieve menstrual discomfort

NUTMEG

Botanical Name: *Myristica aromata, Myristica fragrans, Myristica officinalis*

Family: *Myristicaceae*

The essential oil and CO_2 extract are obtained from the seeds.

Plant Description: Nutmeg is an evergreen tree that grows to a height of about 60 to 100 feet (18 to 30 meters), has large, fragrant dark-green leaves and small yellow flowers that develop into yellow fruit resembling an apricot. The fruit contains a dark-brown seed, which is surrounded by a netlike substance known as mace.

Aromatherapy Uses

Slightly warming; calming, promotes a restful sleep in small amounts, encourages dreaming; mood uplifting, reviving, mental stimulant, improves mental clarity and alertness; improves digestion; loosens tight muscles, relieves aches, pains, sore muscles, and menstrual pains

Precaution

Nutmeg oil can dull the senses. Use small amounts.

ORANGE (BITTER OR SWEET)

Botanical Name: *Citrus aurantium* (*Bitter orange*); *Citrus sinensis* (*Sweet orange*)

Family: *Rutaceae*

The essential oil is obtained from the peel of the fruit.

Plant Description: Orange is an evergreen citrus tree that grows to a height of about 20 to 30 feet (6 to 9 meters) and has fragrant white flowers that develop into edible orange-colored fruit. However, bitter orange is not edible when fresh.

Aromatherapy Uses

Cooling; calming, reduces stress; promotes a restful sleep; mood uplifting; improves mental clarity and alertness; relieves emotional tension and stress, calms angry and irritable children; improves digestion; purifying, helps in the reduction of cellulite; relieves spasms

Precaution

People with dry or sensitive skin may require additional carrier oil when using the essential oil topically. Use small amounts. Orange is phototoxic. Avoid exposure to direct sunlight for several hours after applying the oils on the skin.

PALMAROSA

Botanical Name: *Andropogon martinii, Cymbopogon martinii var. motia*

Family: *Poaceae*

The essential oil is obtained from the plant.

Plant Description: Palmarosa is a fragrant grass that grows to a height of about 9 feet (2.7 meters) and has clusters of flowers that turn red when they mature.

Aromatherapy Uses

Warming, improves circulation; calming, reduces stress; mood uplifting; refreshing; loosens tight muscles; reduces aches, pains, and inflammation; moisturizing and regenerating to the skin; soothes insect bites

PATCHOULI

Botanical Name: *Pogostemon cablin, Pogostemon patchouli*

Family: *Lamiaceae*

The essential oil is obtained from the leaves.

Plant Description: Patchouli is a plant that grows to a height of about 3 feet (0.9 meter), has oblong leaves and whorls of light-purple or lavender flowers.

Aromatherapy Uses

Nerve stimulant; prevents sleep; mood uplifting, euphoric, aphrodisiac; repels insects; healing to the skin; used as a fixative to hold the scent of a fragrance

PEPPERMINT

Botanical Name: *Mentha piperita*

Family: *Lamiaceae*

The essential oil is obtained from the whole plant.

Plant Description: Peppermint is a plant that grows to a height of about 1 to 3 feet (0.3 to 0.9 meter), has a purplish stem and pale-violet flowers.

Aromatherapy Uses

Cooling; vapors open the sinus and breathing passages; mood uplifting, especially for people who have a slow metabolism, aphrodisiac; refreshing, reviving; stimulates the brain, nerves, and metabolism; increases mental clarity, alertness, ability to concentrate, and the memory; sharpens the senses; encourages communication; helps to revive a person from a fainting spell or shock; increases physical strength and endurance; improves digestion, soothes the intestines, relieves flatulence and nausea, increases appetite; freshens bad breath; relieves pain, inflammation, menstrual pain, and cramps; reduces lactation; repels insects, kills parasites; soothes itching skin

Precaution

People with dry or sensitive skin may require additional carrier oil when applying peppermint essential oil topically. Use small amounts. Avoid using before bedtime since the oil can overstimulate the nervous system.

PETITGRAIN

Botanical Name: *Citrus bigaradia*

Family: *Rutaceae*

The essential oil is obtained from the leaves and twigs.

Plant Description: Petitgrain oil is derived from the leaves and twigs of the orange, lemon, or tangerine tree.

Aromatherapy Uses

Cooling; calms the nerves; relieves anxiety, tension, and mental stress; promotes a restful sleep; helpful for meditation; mood uplifting; improves mental clarity, alertness, and the memory; soothes inflamed and irritated skin

PINE

Botanical Name: *Pinus sylvestris*

Family: *Pinaceae*

The essential oil is obtained from the needles and small branches.

Plant Description: Pine is an evergreen tree that grows to a height of about 115 to 130 feet (34.5 to 39 meters), has greenish-blue needle-like leaves and cones.

Aromatherapy Uses

Vapors open the sinus and breathing passages; mood uplifting; refreshing, reviving, stimulates the adrenal glands, promotes vitality; improves mental clarity, alertness, and memory; purifying, removes lymphatic deposits from the body, helps in the reduction of cellulite; lessens pain

Precaution

Pine oil has a strong diuretic effect on the kidneys. Use small amounts with care. People with dry or sensitive skin may require additional carrier oil when applying the essential oil topically.

RAVENSARA AROMATICA

Botanical Name: *Cinnamonum camphora, Ravensara aromatica*

Family: *Lauraceae*

The essential oil is obtained from the leaves.

Plant Description: Ravensara is a small tree that grows to a height of about 60 feet (18 meters), has an anise-scented bark, shiny aromatic green leaves, and green flowers.

Aromatherapy Uses

Calming; reduces stress; vapors open the sinus and breathing passages; deepens the breathing; mood uplifting, refreshing; improves mental clarity; relieves aches and pains

ROSE

Botanical Name: *Rosa centifolia, Rosa damascena*

Family: *Rosaceae*

The essential oil is obtained from the flowers.

Plant Description: There are many varieties of the rose bushes that grow to various heights and produce sweet, fragrant flowers.

Aromatherapy Uses

Cooling; calming, reduces stress, eases emotional shock and grief; mood uplifting, aphrodisiac; increases physical strength; purifying; lessens aches, pains, and inflammation; balances the female hormonal and reproductive system; regenerates skin cells, especially beneficial for dry, sensitive, inflamed, red, aging skin; used for fragrancing

Comments

For the formulas given in this book, it is recommended to use ony the steam distilled rose oil.

ROSEMARY

Botanical Name: *Rosmarinus officinalis*

Family: *Lamiaceae*

The essential oil is obtained from the flowers and leaves.

Plant Description: Rosemary is an aromatic evergreen shrub that grows to a height of about 2 to 6 feet (0.6 to 1.8 meters), has leathery, needle-shaped leaves and small blue flowers. The entire plant is aromatic.

Aromatherapy Uses

Warming, improves circulation; vapors open the sinus and breathing passages; deepens the breathing; mood uplifting, especially for people who have a slow metabolism; stimulating to the metabolism and all other body functions; refreshing; improves mental clarity, alertness, and the memory; improves digestion; purifying, helps in the reduction of cellulite and lymphatic deposits; loosens tight muscles, relieves aches and pains; repels insects

Precaution

Use small amounts. Rosemary oil should be avoided by people prone to epileptic seizures. It is best to avoid using the oil before bedtime due to the stimulating effect.

ROSEWOOD

Botanical Name: *Aniba rosaeodora*

Family: *Lauraceae*

The essential oil is obtained from the bark.

Plant Description: Rosewood is an evergreen tree that grows to a height of about 80 feet (24 meters), has leathery leaves and red flowers.

Aromatherapy Uses

Calming, relieves nervousness and stress; promotes a restful sleep; mood uplifting; lessens pain; regenerates and moisturizes the skin; soothes insect bites

SAGE (SPANISH)

Botanical Name: *Salvia lavandulifolia*

Family: *Lamiaceae*

The essential oil is obtained from the flowers and leaves.

Plant Description: Sage is an evergreen plant that grows to a height of about 2.5 feet (0.75 meter), has aromatic leaves and small purple flowers.

Aromatherapy Uses

Improves circulation; reduces stress; improves alertness; improves digestion; purifying, helps in the reduction of cellulite; relaxes sore muscles; lessens aches, pains, and menstrual pain; strengthening to the body; suppresses perspiration and lactation

Precaution

Spanish sage is less toxic and safer to use than common sage. Both Spanish sage and common sage oils should be avoided by people prone to epileptic seizures.

SANDALWOOD

Botanical Name: *Santalum album*

Family: *Santalaceae*

The essential oil is obtained from the inner wood.

Plant Description: Sandalwood is an evergreen tree that grows to a height of about 30 feet (9 meters), has small purple flowers and small fruits containing a seed.

Aromatherapy Uses

Calming, relaxing, reduces stress; promotes a restful sleep; encourages dreaming; helpful for meditation; soothing to the breathing passages; mood uplifting, euphoric, aphrodisiac; brings out emotions; healing and moisturizing to the skin; used as a fixative to hold the scent of a fragrance

SPEARMINT

Botanical Name: *Mentha spicata, Mentha viridis*

Family: *Lamiaceae*

The essential oil is obtained from the leaves and flowering tops.

Plant Description: Spearmint is a plant that grows to a height of about 1 to 3 feet (0.3 to 0.9 meter), has shiny green leaves, and white or lilac-colored flowers.

Aromatherapy Uses

Cooling; vapors open the sinus and breathing passages; mood uplifting, aphrodisiac; refreshing, reviving, stimulates the metabolism, strengthens the nerves; improves mental clarity, alertness, ability to concentrate, and the memory; sharpens the senses; encourages communication; increases physical strength and endurance; improves digestion, increases the appetite, relieves flatulence, freshens the breath and the intestines; relieves aches, pains, inflammation, and menstrual pain; repels insects; soothes itching skin

Precaution

People with dry or sensitive skin may require additional carrier oil when applying spearmint essential oil topically. Use small amounts. Avoid using before bedtime since the oil can overstimulate the nervous system.

SPIKENARD

Botanical Name: *Nardostachys grandiflora, Nardostachys jatamansi*

Family: *Valerianaceae*

The essential oil is obtained from the roots.

Plant Description: Spikenard is an aromatic plant that grows to a height of about 2 feet (0.6 meter) and has pink bell-shaped flowers.

Aromatherapy Uses

Calming, relaxing, reduces stress; promotes a restful sleep; mood uplifting; reduces inflammation; used as a fixative to hold the scent of a fragrance

SPRUCE

Botanical Name: *Picea mariana*

Family: *Pinaceae*

The essential oil is obtained from the bark and branches.

Plant Description: Spruce is an evergreen tree that grows to a height of about 70 to 200 feet (21 to 60 meters), has blue-green needlelike leaves, red flowers, and purple male and female cones.

Aromatherapy Uses

Calming, reduces stress; vapors open the sinus and breathing passages; deepens the breathing; mood uplifting, euphoric; improves mental clarity; brings out inner feelings; encourages communication

TANGERINE

Botanical Name: *Citrus reticulata*

Family: *Rutaceae*

The essential oil is obtained from the peel of the fruit.

Plant Description: Tangerine is an evergreen citrus tree that grows to a height of about 10 to 25 feet (3 to 7.5 meters) and has fragrant white flowers that develop into edible orange fruit.

Aromatherapy Uses

Cooling; calming, promotes a restful sleep; encourages dreaming; mood uplifting; relieves emotional tension and stress, calms angry and irritable children; improves mental clarity and alertness, sharpens the mind; purifying, helps in the reduction of cellulite

Precaution

People with dry or sensitive skin may require additional carrier oil when using the essential oil topically. Use small amounts. Tangerine is phototoxic. Avoid exposure to direct sunlight for several hours after applying the oil on the skin.

THYME

Botanical Name: *Thymus satureiodes, Thymus vulgaris, Thymus vulgaris var. linalool, Thymus webbianus*

Family: *Lamiaceae*

The essential oil is obtained from the leaves and flowering tops.

Plant Description: Thyme is an evergreen plant that grows to a height of about 1 foot (0.3 meter) and has small leaves and pink or pale lilac-colored flowers.

Aromatherapy Uses

Heating, improves circulation; induces perspiration; relaxes the nerves; vapors open the sinus and breathing passages; mood uplifting; improves mental clarity, alertness, and the memory; sharpens the senses; increases physical endurance and energy; improves digestion, cleanses the intestines; purifying, helps in the reduction of cellulite, waste material, and excessive fluids from the body; loosens tight muscles; relieves aches, pains, inflammation, and spasms; repels insects, kills lice

Comments

The varieties *Thymus satureiodes* and *Thymus vulgaris var. linalool* are less irritating to the skin and less toxic than common thyme.

Precaution

People with dry or sensitive skin may require additional carrier oil when applying thyme essential oil topically. Use small amounts. Thyme should be avoided by people prone to epileptic seizures.

VANILLA

Botanical Name: *Vanilla fragrans, Vanilla planifolia*

Family: *Orchidaceae*

The essential oil is obtained from the pods.

Plant Description: Vanilla is a climbing plant that reaches a height of about 12 feet (3.6 meters) and has clusters of green-yellow flowers followed by aromatic brown seed-pods, containing many small seeds.

Aromatherapy Uses

Calming, reduces stress; promotes a restful sleep; encourages dreaming; mood uplifting, aphrodisiac; fragrancing; used as a fixative to hold the scent of a fragrance

Comments

For the formulas in this book, it is recommended that vanilla CO_2 extracted oil be used.

VETIVER

Botanical Name: *Andropogon muricatus, Vetiveria zizanoides*

Family: *Poaceae*

The essential oil is obtained from the roots.

Plant Description: Vetiver is a tropical grass that grows to a height of about 4 to 8 feet (1.2 to 2.4 meters), has sharp-edged leaves, tiny flowers, and aromatic roots.

Aromatherapy Uses

Calms nervousness, relieves stress and tension; promotes a restful sleep; mood uplifting; strengthens the body; improves digestion; loosens tight muscles, relieves pain; healing to the skin; repels insects; used as a fixative to hold the scent of a fragrance

YLANG-YLANG

Botanical Name: *Cananga odorata var. genuina*

Family: *Annonaceae*

The essential oil is obtained from the flowers.

Plant Description: Ylang-ylang is an evergreen tree that grows to a height of about 80 to 100 feet (24 to 30 meters), has glossy leaves and large yellow fragrant flowers that develop into black fruit containing many seeds.

Aromatherapy Uses

Calming, relaxing, reduces stress; promotes a restful sleep; mood uplifting, euphoric, aphrodisiac; brings out feelings, enhances communication; loosens tight muscles; lessens pain

Index

About the Authors

David Schiller and **Carol Schiller** are the authors of seven internationally published books on the use of essential oils, and cofounders of the International Aromatherapy and Herb Association (IAHA). Since 1986, David and Carol have been studying and researching the benefits of plant oils, and determining their practical uses and applications. They have been instructing classes and training workshops for companies, colleges, and other educational organizations since 1989. Carol has been a featured presenter at international conferences.